PRAISE FOR

# WAR STORIES

FROM THE FORGOTTEN SOLDIERS

"In his compelling book, Dr. Beal opens our eyes to the psychological aftermath of war. We certainly owe our men and women in uniform a great deal of gratitude for their sacrifices. But, equally as important, I believe we also owe them a greater understanding of what they face upon returning home. This book, rooted in first-hand accounts by service members, is that source for greater understanding and compassion."

—**SENATOR BOB DOLE,** World War II veteran

"In a word, it is BRILLIANT. I have never read anything quite like it. The way [Dr. Beal combines] factual information (from a multitude of authors and sources), clinical observations, story-telling, personal observations, and reflections is as unique as it is engaging."

—**ROBERT KOFFMAN, MD,** Navy Captain, former Director for Psychological Health to the Navy Surgeon General, Former Deputy Director of Clinical Operations at the National Intrepid Center of Excellence in Bethesda, Maryland

"Dr. Beal's background gives him an unique perspective, having both empathy as a fellow soldier during his service [as a physician during the Vietnam war] as well as professional objectivity as a civilian psychiatrist treating soldiers from the Iraq-Afghanistan war. In this remarkable collection of riveting stories and thought-provoking reflections, Dr. Beal shares his decades of experience observing and counseling the 1% of our population who bear the untold burden of protecting our country. He challenges readers to learn how to ask our veterans about their service, listen to their stories and their ongoing challenges, and become more compassionately aware of the immeasurable cost of war on our military members, their families, and the society surrounding them. This extraordinary book is an emotionally and academically charged call to action for service members and civilians alike!"

—**PETER S. COOKE,** Major General (Ret.) US Army Reserve; former Director of National Center for Veterans' Studies; former Chairman of Army Reserve Forces Policy Committee

"In *War Stories From the Forgotten Soldiers,* Dr. Edward W. Beal chronicles his treatment of traumatized GIs. Whether it's killing a young boy who was probably just curious, targeting and killing people daily and endlessly from a TV screen, wanting to take out all your anger and grief on a loved one, or some other episodic absurdity of the detritus of endless, meaningless war, Beal has probed the problems. In all, Beal's most telling point, among several dozens of searing revelations, is this: 'Sharing in the soldier's moral grief is not just a national duty; rather, it is a moral obligation that citizens owe to soldiers who fought in their place.' Quite needless to say, however, the obligatory 'Thank you for your service', rendered daily by countless Americans, doesn't pass muster. But Beal tells us repeatedly what does. Few of us are listening though; sadly, far fewer of us could do it even if we were."

—**LAWRENCE WILKERSON,** Colonel, US Army (Ret.), Chief of Staff to Secretary of State Colin Powell (2002–2005), Special Assistant to Powell when Chairman of the Joint Chiefs of Staff (1989–1993), and Deputy Director and Director of the USMC War College (1993–1997). Visiting Professor of Government and Public Policy at the College of William & Mary

"Some 99% of Americans have little contact with the military today. Because very few know anything of the experiences or consequences for those who serve, deploying them becomes even easier. In *War Stories* Dr. Ted Beal, who has spent years meeting with soldiers and confronting with them the horrors they have faced and the memories they endure, asks us all to confront them. With powerful accounts and candid observations, he tells stories that need to be heard by all citizens, especially by those who send the young to war."

—**JAMES WRIGHT,** President Emeritus of Dartmouth College, Historian, former Marine, Author of *Enduring Vietnam: An American Generation and Its War.*

"Most Americans patronizingly refer to every member of their military as a hero while looking away from the physical and emotional scars of these broken heroes. Dr. Beal forces us to hear and see them."

—**DENNIS LAICH,** Major General (Ret.) US Army, Co-Founder, All-Volunteer Force Forum

"This book captivated me intellectually and emotionally. I could not put it down! Dr. Beal's detailed accounts of his stunningly candid conversations with returning and deploying soldiers gives us a window into the trauma and hidden-from-plain-view suffering of those who fight in wars. I learned not only about the soldiers, but about myself, my ignorance regarding the costs of modern warfare and my responsibility as a citizen and leader to move beyond polite gratitude when interacting with returning soldiers. Here is a work every American should read, regardless of political persuasion, economic circumstance, race or culture. It's a rare, real and gripping book that will moisten your eyes and enlighten your mind."

—**JOHN J. ENGELS,** President Leadership Coaching, Inc., Rochester, New York

"The well-intentioned 'Thank you for your service' may seem short-sighted after reading this powerful and sobering insight into the trauma of war inflicted on our country's volunteer warriors who willingly step into unknown physical and mental dangers on behalf of a mostly unaware civilian population. Ted Beal examines this paradox through a prism of five decades of providing psychotherapy, including seven years helping service members and their families face and overcome emotional withdrawal. His series of moving essays about traumatized service members puts into startling context their experiences and the effect on marriages, family bonds and seemingly simple relationships within military and civilian communities. Listening and learning are the keys to understanding how to help these service members. Reading this book is a necessary first step."

—**CAPTAIN TIMOTHY J. GORMAN,** US Navy (Ret.)

"Beal's book helps us understand the sacrifice of soldiers when we think about using force for 'national security reasons.' I recommend it as required reading for anyone who considers war a legitimate policy option to deal with perceived threats to national security."

—**ROBERT L. GALLUCCI, PHD,** Former President, John D. and Catherine T. MacArthur Foundation, Former Assistant Secretary of State for Political-Military Affairs, Former Deputy Executive Chairman of the United Nations Special Commission overseeing the disarmament of Iraq, Professor and Former Dean, Georgetown University School of Foreign Service; Former Director of the John W. Kluge Center at the Library of Congress

"'War and killing, guilt and grief are far too important not to be shared' writes Dr. Edward Beal. In his *War Stories From the Forgotten Soldiers*, Beal calls on each of us to listen, feel, care and reach out to the four million veterans who served our country these past twenty years. The stories he heard over the past eight years are gripping, full of trauma and suffering. Our role is clear: engage with the 1 percent who volunteer, extend love and respect, and help each other come together. This book inspires us to heal in every way."

—**AMBASSADOR FREDERICK D. BARTON,** Author of *Peace Works*, first Assistant Secretary of State for Conflict and Stabilization Operations; Lecturer and Co-Director, Scholars in the Nation's Service Initiative (SINSI), Woodrow Wilson School—Princeton University

"There are many books about the wars in this century filled with platitudes. One of the many virtues of this one is that it moves beyond 'Thank you for your service' to the complexities of being or treating a Soldier or Marine in the Long War since 9/11.

"Dr Beal treated those with both physical and mental health issues from the Long War at Walter Reed National Military Medical Center for nearly eight years. Walter Reed has borne the lion's share on the severely wounded for the last eighteen plus wars.

"As a psychiatrist who served 28 years in the Army, including many years at Walter Reed, I especially liked the section on 'Recruiting: A Necessary Task', where Dr Beal comes face to face with the moral and ethical dilemmas of recruiting young men and women to serves in today's amorphous battlefields.

"This is not only required reading for mental health providers who work with the Veteran and Service Member population; it should be required for all providers."

—**ELSPETH CAMERON RITCHIE, MD, MPH,** Colonel, US Army (Ret.); Chair of Psychiatry, Medstar Washington Hospital Center

"Americans now generally know that many service members sustain wounds that are not visible. In the past decade and a half, phrases like 'traumatic brain injury' (TBI) and 'post-traumatic stress syndrome' (PTSD) have entered the national lexicon. Growing familiarity with these and related conditions encourages the public to think not only about what might be done for those suffering but also about the hidden costs of military conflict. But I suspect that the understanding of many concerned citizens is limited simply because until now no one has published for a general audience detailed descriptions and expert analyses of actual cases. Dr. Edward Beal's excellent book fills this void. Drawing on his experience in more than 5,000 sessions with injured service members, Dr. Beal discusses the conditions of more than thirty of the patients he has treated. The clarity and compassion with which he writes will leave an indelible impression on all who read this important book."

—**JUDGE GREGORY E. MAGGS,** US Court of Appeals for the Armed Forces (Colonel, US Army, Ret.)

"Read this book to learn to listen to the veteran in your life. Dr. Ted Beal provides a moving personal account on the importance of veterans' stories as a means of individual healing, insight for those who know and love veterans and inspiration for our nation to embrace the values and valor of those who volunteer to serve our country."

—**BOB PATRICK,** Colonel, US Army (Ret.); former Director, Veterans History Project, Library of Congress

"Edward Beal has written the book you didn't know you were missing—about the men and women in uniform that war ruins for peace. It took courage and dedication to listen for seven years to their stories, their lives, the way war crushed their spirit. As Dr. Beal learned, they don't want to hear 'thank you for your service.' They want to be heard. In *War Stories* they are, loud, clear and heart-breaking."

—**PHYLLIS THEROUX,** Author

". . . *War Stories from the Forgotten Soldiers* . . . is such a moving and eloquent book, and I am quite in awe of its scope and depth. To me it has two stories that are inseparable: one of the soldiers overwhelmed by their combat experience and seeking help, the other of your own return to meaningful and engaging work after retirement. It begins in the trenches of psychiatric encounter, then zooms out to consider institutional history of the teleprovider unit and ultimately how to reconcile the dual morality of war and peace. The framework of classical literature reminds us that the problem of warriors re-entering the civil community is a human universal—perpetual intergroup conflict matched with perpetual remorse. I can imagine [Dr. Beal] Skyping an interview with Odysseus after he had come home and massacred half the population of Ithaca for partying with his wife.

"I felt the reality of those military personnel as if they were in the room... [The] chapter structure with each individual personal contact followed by professional reflection brings a nice balance between interpersonal intensity and urgency, then quiet rumination on what it means. [Dr. Beal] shows the inner agony and bewilderment on the other side of the legendary competence of US military personnel.

"The book is coming at the right time, with the word 'forgotten' in the title. The whole Trump spectacle has distracted us from the 9/11 wars before we had a chance to understand them. The result is a forgotten generation of service members in an isolated caste, often forced to call attention to their existence through self-destruction. Here in Maine even with our small population, there were 29 military suicides in 2016, which rose to 48 in 2017, so rather than subsiding, the problem seems to increase as the wars themselves recede from national attention.

"I hope this book gets the wide audience it deserves. It is humane and eloquent and I feel enlightened and changed by reading it. It illuminates the darkness that I was groping [through] in the novel with the light of experience and reason..."

—**WILLIAM CARPENTER,** Professor Emeritus, College of the Atlantic, Author of *The Wooden Nickel*

"Edward Beal's book, *War Stories From the Forgotten Soldiers*, is both riveting and very important. The book clearly delineates the key changes in the US military in a single generation: from a draft Army to a volunteer Army, from many soldiers to one percent of our population protecting us, and the evolution of highly specialized, frequently heart-rending jobs that the modern soldier must perform.

This has led us to a virtually complete disassociation between today's soldier and the civilian world where many/most of us no longer know or relate to recent or current enlisted men and women.

"Beal argues that we, as a society, must do more than 'thank them for their service.' We should actively engage with soldiers and veterans, work with them in our jobs, socialize with them after work, and befriend them in all aspects of their and our lives. If we fail to do this, the great schism that has now been created between the American soldier and the American public may become irreconcilable. In fact, that schism may have already occurred."

—**HENRY SONDHEIMER, MD,** Professor Emeritus of Pediatrics (Cardiology), University of Colorado SOM, Former Associate Dean for Admissions, University of Colorado SOM, Former Senior Director of Medical Education, Association of American Medical Colleges (AAMC)

"An authentic narrative meditation on telepsychiatry's power to enable a shared treatment journey for patient and psychiatrist. An important education to better understand how telepsychiatry enhances access to care and connects us across distance."

—**JAY H. SHORE, MD, MPH,** Professor Department of Psychiatry and Family Medicine, and Director of Telemedicine, Helen and Arthur E Johnson Depression Center, University of Colorado, Anschutz Medical Campus

"These are compelling, moving and well-written stories from the perspective of a compassionate and seasoned psychiatrist. This book provides a valuable guide for the civilian mental health practitioner who will be working with veterans, soldiers or their families."

—**STEVEN A. EPSTEIN, MD,** Physician Executive Director, MedStar Behavioral Health, Professor and Chair of Psychiatry, Georgetown University School of Medicine and MedStar Georgetown University Hospital, past President of the Academy of Psychosomatic Medicine.

"Dr. Beal has brought a lifetime of clinical experience to working with US soldiers and veterans. His ability to listen, advocate, and communicate with them and us is a gift. Dr. Beal's moving prose brings their narratives to light in a way that allows us to better understand their heroic sacrifices and struggles and encourages us to give voice to their need for improved personal and institutional support and resources. It's a fabulous book. How moving!!!"

—**LIZA H. GOLD, MD,** Board-Certified Forensic Psychiatrist, President Elect (Oct 2019) American Academy of Psychiatry and the Law; Clinical Professor of Psychiatry, Georgetown University School of Medicine

"Someone who has not served in the military will find in this book a new respect for the courage and fortitude of those who have served. This book, written with the personal goal of being as objective as possible, does not evoke pity as much as it does respect. It does not bring about sympathy as much as it does regard for the character that underlies sacrifice in the line of duty.

"Ted Beal, with the practiced eye of the clinical psychiatrist, reaches beyond the clinical to present real stories of men and women in the military who have experienced considerable pain, suffering, and disability in the line of duty. The impact is enormous in depth, scope, and intensity. These stories inevitably will make a difference to the reader, far beyond other accounts of experiences of war and service."

—**SCOTTY HARGROVE, PHD,** ABPP Former Professor of Psychology and Chair, Department of Psychology, University of Mississippi, Past President, American Orthopsychiatric Association

"In offering us *War Stories From the Forgotten Soldiers,* the author invites us to hear various morally and emotionally distorted world views from dedicated patriots whose psychic wounds have them struggling to keep their very souls alive. Author Beal is most compelling in his closing observation that 'Knowing a soldier personally is perhaps the most powerful intervention of all,' and in his plea to the reader: 'America needs you.' Read this book."

—**J.R. QUIRK,** Author, *Compassionate Warrior—A Memoir*

"Based on extensive interviews, Edward W. Beal's *War Stories from Forgotten Soldiers* explores with empathy the impact that combat had on his patients. He delineates the stress, trauma, and pain borne by the relatively small number of men and women who have experienced war firsthand. They still grapple with their memories of the harsh reality of combat. This thoughtful, sensitive book is highly recommended."

—**RICHARD HUNT,** Author of *Pacification, The American Struggle for Vietnam's Hearts and Minds,* Former Director of the Oral History Program at the US Army Center of Military History

"Every person has a life story, comprised of many life-altering experiences—both tragic and joyous, and both mundane and profound. In the annals of memorable historical and fictional accounts of the impact of war on human lives, it is commonly concluded that war never really resolves any conflicts and only serves to create next generations of human suffering and vendetta conflicts. Yet, there are invariably lessons to be learned and taught during and after each war, so as to promote human quality of life and future peace.

"Joining the pantheon of truly important commentaries about the human casualties of war and attempts at recovery is a new publication, *War Stories From the Forgotten Soldiers.*

"In this moving, poignant, personal and powerful book, Dr. Beal recounts many of the memorable conversations, emotional reactions, and insights gained with several of his Iraq and Afghanistan combat veteran patients at Walter Reed Army Medical Center from 2010 to 2017. While there are no new revelations about the typical psychological, social, physical, occupational, and spiritual consequences that persons such as these brave women and men have suffered, Dr. Beal goes well beyond previously published war tomes, as he and his patients invite the reader into the sanctuary of healing at a major military treatment facility. In offering the reader the personal opportunity to observe the art of psychotherapy, he also provides unique insights into the deeper and broader war injuries to the communities in which these veterans and their families reside. In doing so, he challenges each reader to 'get to know' military service members and 'listen to their stories,' since 'our country owes it to them.'

"As the individual soldier stories in each chapter are so gripping and Dr. Beal's thoughts are so intriguing, so this book will be hard for any reader to put down until it is finished. Dr. Beal facilitates the easy-read content with an excellent chapter organization and a conversational writing style. He soon seems not only like a highly caring and compassionate person, but a psychiatrist whom anyone would want to enlist to help work through a crisis, conflict, trauma, or personal suffering. The reader is allowed to see him as a deeply feeling, highly experienced, practical, and insightful clinician whose shared goal with each patient and family is comforting and healing, even when curing is not possible. Dr. Beal also adroitly and convincingly provides numerous relevant and informative citations about effective psychological coping techniques, psychiatric epidemiology, other authors' observations about war-related outcomes for humans, and the complex moral and political aspects of recent, past, and likely future wars.

"While some authors might dance around or superficially reflect upon the deeper societal and moral issues that have impacted him and his patients, he thoughtfully, objectively, and honestly lays them out as one of the foundations of the book. He also crafts unique discussions about the socio-political aspects of military recruiting and the critical roles of social institutional leadership in the adequate planning and provision of essential long-term programs to assist war veterans and their families with their initial and enduring health, social, and disability needs.

This important new book should be recommended reading for (1) all mental health and health care professionals who provide clinical services to veterans; (2) those who employ and supervise combat veterans; (3) all federal, legislative and executive branch leaders who plan, budget, and execute wars; and (4) any citizen who wants to better understand the common personal struggles and triumphs of combat veterans. It should also be required reading for (1) all mental health professional trainees and their supervisors; (2) all military service academy students and faculty members; and (3) all students and faculty at military war colleges, command and general staff schools, and all non-commissioned officer training programs. As each reader is able to better comprehend the salient lessons in this book offered by Dr. Beal and his brave patients, so he or she will be better prepared to join combat veterans in becoming 'twice a citizen.'"

—**ALEX RODRIGUEZ, MD,** Captain, US Navy (Ret.), and Staff Psychiatrist, Bay Pines VA Health Care System (Florida)

"Service to the country in the military, especially in wartime, is stressful at best, traumatic and devastating at worst. Ted brings the costs of these experiences to the reader in brilliant detail. One is reminded of *All Quiet on the Western Front*, when the consequences of war are inescapable."

—**LARRY PIFER,** Army Veteran; Engineer, Johns Hopkins University Applied Physics Laboratory

". . . [These] essays are a hard read—not an easy one, but a meaningful one . . ."

—**CRAIG DORMAN,** RDML, USN (Ret.) and PhD.

"Wow! What an incredible book . . . I was riveted, and it made me feel compelled, as a citizen, to take the type of action [Dr. Beal advises]. . . . [My] father is a Vietnam veteran, so I understand some of the stories and revelations . . . but I learned a great deal, too."

—**CHERYL ROSS,** Editor

*War Stories from the Forgotten Soldiers:*
*Listen As They Speak*

by Edward W. Beal



ISBN 978-1-63393-947-9

LCCN: TXu 2-161-711



Published by

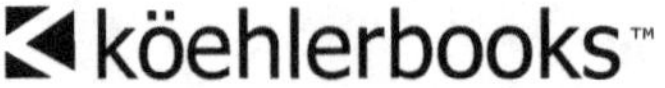

210 60th Street
Virginia Beach, VA 23451
800–435–4811
www.koehlerbooks.com

# WAR STORIES

## FROM THE FORGOTTEN SOLDIERS

***Listen As They Speak***

To Carol and Dennis,

**EDWARD W. BEAL**

In appreciation of our long and enduring friendship

Ted

VIRGINIA BEACH
CAPE CHARLES

# AUTHOR'S NOTE

The sessions related in this book occurred while I was working in telepsychiatry at Walter Reed Army Medical Center from March 2010 to August 2017. I wrote about the events as I was experiencing them. Since they were written at various times, I periodically reintroduce myself to maintain continuity in the essays

The views expressed herein are those of the author and do not necessarily reflect the official policy or position of the Department of the Army, Navy, Air force, Department of Defense, Department of Veterans Affairs nor the US Government.

Name, rank, locations and some specific characteristics of soldiers have been changed to protect their identity.

The author used the term PTSD instead of PTS, preferred by many service members. PTSD is used in the practice of psychiatry. The author in no way means to disrespect the wishes of service members by adding the D for "disorder."

The author used the words "soldier" and "service member" interchangeably. Although the author interviewed a number of sailors, airmen and women, and Marines, the use of soldier as an inclusive noun is for the convenience of the general reader and not meant to disrespect the service of those men and women who served in other branches of the service besides the Army.

*To the service members and their families whose experiences made these stories possible*

*and to Joe Bradley, whose encouragement and efforts made their publication a reality.*

# TABLE OF CONTENTS

# PRELUDE

Not long after I began working with service members via telehealth, I realized that these men and women were as emotionally important to me as my work was for them. I soon learned that the sessions were stressful; I had to speak with others about what I was hearing. I was unable to listen and contain their suffering inside myself. I had to get it out.

When I came home from work, I was so emotionally spent that sometimes I went to bed—something I had never done in my professional career. Most days, I spoke with my wife. She encouraged me to keep talking and tell others about the work. A friend asked if I would write an essay about a service member's experience. I sent the essay to his publication, the *Catholic Peace Fellowship Newsletter* in Philadelphia. It was well received, and he asked for a second essay. A month later, I was a "regular" in the quarterly.

Writing made me a better listener. The more I wrote about the experiences, I learned I did not have to talk as much in order to hear. I found it was important to be calm and honest. When I had no idea how to respond to a tragic story, I replied directly to the service member, "I have never heard anything like this before, and I do not know what to say." Service members talked, in part, because they knew I was listening and asking questions. The more calmly I could speak, the more they could explain their experience. It was a bit of a tightrope trying to never go beyond what the service member could manage emotionally or what I could manage as well.

Some sessions were so stressful that I could not wait to go home and speak with my wife. I would exit my office, take two steps, knock on the door of the psychiatrist next to me, sit down, and say, "I have to talk to you about what I just heard." After a few minutes of sharing the experience with another human being, I could go back to see the next service member. I realized that the listening, the talking, and the writing were helping the soldier I was treating. The more I was able to write and talk about their stories, the more they were able to talk about their experiences. I grew to understand the truth behind why speaking about misunderstood problems improved by discussing them. Grief and trauma can become a collective experience rather than just be contained within an individual.

I encouraged service members to write their stories. Many have done so, especially with one another. They protest that they do not want to share their stories with their spouses or any civilians. They desire to protect others from their trauma. While their motivation to protect is understandable and laudable, it is important to move beyond that. War and killing, guilt and grief are far too important not to be shared with willing listeners.

I wrote these essays to help service members, with the hope that the essays will inspire readers to get to know a service member and his or her story. Unless our civilians help manage the service member's trauma, then those who fought in our stead will carry all the grief and anguish for our country. That neglect from civilians would be the ultimate moral betrayal. Our country owes it to service members and to ourselves to share the service members' trauma as we confront and contemplate continuous war.

# INTRODUCTION

The chairman of the Department of Psychiatry at Walter Reed Army Medical Center was giving a lecture about the war in Iraq and Afghanistan. As I listened, I found myself tearful as he spoke informatively and factually, giving little hint at the carnage war produces. Later, as I attempted to ask questions, trying to find a way to offer my assistance to soldiers, I choked up and had difficulty speaking.

In 2008, I did not understand what I was experiencing. Now, after working for nearly eight years with servicemen and women, I believe I was then unconsciously aware of what I am now consciously aware: Those men and women who have been deploying to Iraq and Afghanistan and returning carry the suffering and grief of a nation's nearly twenty years of continuous war.

Just hearing those cold, hard facts within the lecture about the numbers of service members going and coming had managed to touch my heart. Now in my present work, watching these multihandicapped service members piece their lives back together, the unspoken grief is omnipresent and everywhere. The soldiers emotionally compartmentalized their experience of killing in order to survive. So, have Americans as a group compartmentalized our war effort in order to avoid the pain of understanding what we have done and are doing? We owe it to our servicemen and women, our national duty, to make a collective effort to understand.

Americans fail to understand what even the ancient Greeks knew was critical to the preservation of their society and democracy. The collective narrative experience, the telling of the story by the traumatized soldier to a trustworthy audience, the collective experiencing of terror, rage, and grief, is critical to regain the soul of the individual and the integrity of our society.

Homer's *Iliad* and the *Odyssey*, the oldest known books on war, chronicle not only the battle but the return of the soldiers and reintegration into society. Aristotle "made tragedy the centerpiece of education for citizens in a democracy. In *Achilles in Vietnam: Combat Trauma and the Undoing of Character*, Jonathan Shay shows how Sophocles' plays manifested the belief that the communal experience of tragedies was central to meaningful human existence. Bryan Doerries (2017), director of Theater of War Productions, said, "Ancient Greek drama appears to have been an elaborate ritual aimed at helping combat veterans return to civilian life after deployments during a century that saw 80 years of war."

America has a national duty to collectively understand the burden that should not be retained by the 1 percent who serve. Our failure to understand and communicate with one another over the past fifty years has contributed to a form of tribalism that divides our citizens. A national conversation between civilians and soldiers, our warrior tribe, could lead us, paradoxically, out of our tribalism to a common ground of national service. We might actually answer the question so eloquently inferred by President Kennedy: "Ask not what your country can do for you, ask what you can do for your country."

Read these essays, start your journey, and think about what awaits you. The more Americans who reach out to the marginalized 1 percent who keep us safe, the more we might recognize our common humanity and destiny, our common ground. Learning about their courage may give us courage and connectedness. We need their help as much as they need ours.

What more is there to learn about war and the soldiers who fight? How important is it to know what soldiers do? What is involved in knowing a service member personally or his or her family? Is it important to understand why wars are started and why he or she fights? What is it that keeps us from having that conversation? The Greeks understood that from sharing tragedy arises the bond of mutual human experience. Service members want to know their mission. Our citizenry must understand war and their experience before deciding which wars we want to fight. As citizens, the answers to these questions carry the seeds of our national common ground.

Most of us do not personally know these current heroes or their stories. In fact, research finds that "71 per cent of Americans say they do not understand the problems faced by those who have served since 9/11" (Military Service Initiative from the Bush Center—bushcenter.org). In this same source, veterans report that "the public has 'little awareness' of the issues facing them and their families."

I believe that regardless of one's view about war or how it began, citizens have a moral duty to care for and understand those who volunteered to serve on the country's behalf.

Many of us have had the experience described by essayist Pete Candler in a 2017 Veterans Day article for *The Washington Post* in which his father volunteered for service in the controversial Vietnam War. Candler said that his father "never once volunteered to talk about it." Candler wrote, *"I wish he would tell me about it himself."* By the end of the essay, Candler admits what "I actually meant but did not have the guts to say: *I wish I had the courage to ask.*"

If we did ask, we might get the answer provided by Capt. Jerry Yellin. He flew the last combat mission of World War II with the Seventy-eighth Fighter Squadron. At age ninety-three he said, "The sounds and sights of war never leave you. . . . Well, it's never over. When you've been in combat, it just plain is never over." He went on to say, "You can emulate the sights, the sounds of war. You can never ever emulate the smell of 28,000 bodies in the sun in Iwo Jima" (Eltagouri, 2017).

"The feeling that one has when a buddy dies," Yellin added. "You just can't emulate that. We have a burden civilians will never understand." With more than seventy years of perspective on World War II, he now says, "We have to understand that killing for what you believe is the heart of evil. And it still goes on. We are all human beings together. I'm representing hopefully, humbly, honestly the 16 million I served with in World War II."

That is an answer that is not easy to hear.

If we did ask and listen, we might hear the advice of a "wise old retired Marine colonel" quoted by Robert Killebrew in *Foreign Policy*. "So you want to be a career soldier? Good for you. But remember that the longer you stay in uniform, the less you will really understand about the country you protect. Democracy is the antithesis of the military life; it's chaotic, dishonest, disorganized, and at the same time glorious, exhilarating, and free—which you are not.

"After a while, if you stay in, you'll be tempted to say 'Look you civilians, we've got a better way. We're better organized. We're patriotic, and we know what it is to sacrifice. Be like us.' And you'll be dead wrong, son. If you're a career soldier, you may defend democracy, but you won't understand it or be a part of it. What's more, you'll always be a stranger to your own society. That's the sacrifice you'll be making."

So, are these men and women who serve and protect us condemned to being strangers in their homeland? Are they shunned and consigned to being misunderstood by all of us?

This book recounts my experience of learning about war by way of listening to soldiers and writing essays and sketches that convey their, and their families,' experiences with war. Following each essay are brief professional thoughts and questions generated by each soldier's experience. An overall goal is to generate discussion, first among those of us who are uninvolved in war. Later, these stories may generate further discussion and listening between those uninvolved and those who serve to protect us.

I hope that this book will expand your understanding of the experience of war, clarify your personal position about war, and help you be more comfortable speaking with soldiers and families who are fighting our wars. Learning about their courage may give us courage and connectedness. We need their help as much as they need ours.

## SETTING THE SCENE

My career in medicine, my first job, was as a captain in the Army. Now, some fifty years later near the end of my career, I again work with soldiers. In 1967, President Lyndon Johnson sent a letter drafting me into the US Army, telling me I was to arrive at Tan Son Nhut Air Base wearing khakis and combat boots. A long path led me instead to the Medical Field Service School at Fort Sam Houston, Texas. My job was teaching medical colleagues the diagnosis and treatment of tropical diseases in soldiers serving in Vietnam. I served for two years but had no direct exposure to combat. Although I did not agree with the war effort (and had thought about being a conscientious objector), I am proud of my service and I am pleased that I did it.

As a part of "my duties," my wife was invited to tea at the home of the commanding general. Meeting his wife for the first time, my wife asked what her husband did. She replied, "He is the CO of the base." My wife said, "Oh, my husband tried to be a conscientious objector also." I am happy to report our marriage survived, but it was "tough sledding" for a while.

Some of my soldier trainees were former medical school classmates. They knew I had no more experience than they did. During a very formal lecture I had to give to 500 officers/physicians, a former classmate disrespectfully yelled from the back of the room, "Hey, Ted, how many cases of malaria have you really seen?" The Army had coached me to say somewhat fewer than 100, the officially reported number diagnosed in the United States. Now, nearing the end of my career, I have a two-day-a-week job in telepsychiatry at Walter Reed Army Medical Center (WRAMC). I see fifteen to twenty soldiers a week, probably about four to 5,000 service member visits so far. Many are on their way to Iraq or Afghanistan or have just returned from deployment. Some have been deployed four or five times.

Sometimes, I think this work is a curious path for a physician who explored being a conscientious objector during the Vietnam War. I have my reservations about all these wars but have no reservations about helping soldiers. I help make decisions as to whether soldiers are suitable for returning to combat. Do those decisions indicate that I am contributing to the war effort?

As I watched my colleagues go and return from Vietnam, they, like the entire American society, were changed by the experience. Many societal observers believe the lingering effects of the Vietnam War are a major factor in the partisan divide currently experienced by Americans. Citizens learned that they cannot always trust their government to do the right thing nor to be truthful about its actions. Antipathy about the war led citizens to protest but also to inappropriately treat returning soldiers negatively. Some citizens blamed the military for the war. Continuing the war was divisive, but citizens then were intensely involved with one another and with the military.

War today is different, more technological, and fought with fewer people. It involves more sophisticated weaponry and fewer deaths but more physical and psychological traumas in survivors. By further contrast, today only 1 percent of society—soldiers serving in Iraq and Afghanistan and their families—are carrying the burden of these wars. Approximately 99 percent of us appear virtually unaffected as we watch the war and know little about it.

Our collective "war effort" resides in a small number of citizen soldiers who defend our honor, our way of life, and contain our ongoing anxiety and unshared grief about the moral and physical trauma. Most of us do not personally know these current heroes or their stories. Society as a whole has partitioned the war effort into this highly trained technologically sophisticated small group whose job is to fight our wars. This situation was not always so.

During prior wars, 75 percent of us had an immediate family member in uniform. During the Iraq and Afghanistan wars, few Americans are close to someone with military experience. Previously, the common draft brought citizens from all sections of society together for the purpose of serving. True, there was a lot of jockeying for deferments. We could, however, criticize the military during the Vietnam War because they were *us* and we had personal knowledge of who the military was.

Now, our unfamiliarity with soldiers feeds our heroic worship and gratitude for those who fight our wars. We love the troops, but we would rather not think about them beyond "thank you for your service." In other words, "Welcome back, but please keep your experience to yourself."

This distant heroic relationship between citizen and soldier is not the American tradition. The current nature of this relationship creates a sense of elitism that poorly serves both citizen and soldier. Elitism and distance lead to unrealistic treatment of soldiers by society. Sebastian Junger in his book *Tribe: On Homecoming and Belonging* has suggested that the nature of our society—the way it is organized and the loss of closeness—is one of the reasons that the incidence of post-traumatic stress disorder (PTSD) is so high in our soldiers. Our heroic distant relationship also makes it more difficult to understand how to integrate soldiers back into society once their term of service ends.

When soldiers and citizens come from the same neighborhood or same family or same area, a much more balanced approach to war ensues. Sending your son or daughter or your neighbor off to war, rather than a stranger, *does* make a difference. If the nation's warriors were our children, we would know some of the facts about their service. We would know that four million veterans have served since 9/11 and that large numbers of these men and women are transitioning back to civilian life. If they served in combat, they had a 52 percent chance of having an emotionally traumatic experience. While serving, there was a 60 percent chance that one of their peers would be badly injured and a 47 percent chance that one of their peers would be killed while serving (Bush Center).

Those are the percentages, but the actual numbers are more concrete. One survey (*Huffington Post,* 2015) says that 6,845 Americans were killed and over 900,000 injured in Iraq and Afghanistan. The 111,000 Afghans were estimated to have been killed directly and indirectly up to 360,000—to date. Iraqi civilians killed are estimated from as low as 110,000 to as high as 1.2 million (*Huffington Post,* 2017).

Since our medical and surgical skills have improved significantly, those who are wounded do not die as often on the battlefield. More soldiers survive after injury than in previous wars. With survival comes significant physical and psychological injuries; for example, 1,700 soldiers lost one or more limbs while serving. Over 380,000 suffer traumatic brain injury (Defense and Veteran Brain Injury Center). A RAND study reports "at least 20 percent of Iraq and Afghanistan veterans have PTSD and/or Depression" (Veterans Statistics, 2015). We are only beginning to recognize the moral trauma.

The choice to go to war, the manner in which wars are fought, and the ability to absorb the subsequent suffering "depends on society's answer to the question, 'Whose children will go?'" (Fallows, 1980)

It is a fact that 99 percent of us can say, "Not our children."

Our society will suffer so long as we fail to know those who serve and their experiences. Our discussions about who we are as a nation and our decisions about when and where we will go to war will never be honest as long as we have scapegoats to serve, no matter how heroic their service (Fallows, 1980).

Moral clarity, clearly reasoned and understood, goes a long way toward mitigating the suffering caused by war and killing. In his *Washington Post* article "At Last, Afghans on the Front Lines," David Ignatius wrote of the intensity of these differences—about whose children will fight and whether they should go to war—as well as how political differences disappear when you are both defending the same foxhole.

For the last few years, I have watched these two new wars. I read a lot about the war, debated its merits, and viewed a weekly list of names and photos on TV. I didn't know anything about these service members and their experiences—those men and women who give their lives in service to our country. Opportunities over the years to give an hour a week in my private office taking care of soldiers passed me by. Like many of my colleagues, I declined, feeling that a single person in a private office was ill equipped for the task.

Then in 2009, an opportunity to work in telepsychiatry at Walter Reed Army Medical Center came my way. A new clinic based at Walter Reed was designed to treat soldiers all over the United Sates, and maybe the globe, via closed circuit telecommunications.

The complexity of clearing the security and competence hurdles is hard to exaggerate. More than three months of time and countless emails, letters, and phone calls were required. Once hired, it took an equal amount of time to complete Army educational programs and become credentialed at military bases throughout the United States. I actually started the job in March 2010.

Walter Reed is an impressive organization. It is certainly a government bureaucracy, but after *The Washington Post* exposé on soldier treatment a few years ago, leaders hired a top executive from Disney World. His job was to teach the Walter Reed community about graciousness, courtesy, and hospitality. After six months, so impressed with his Walter Reed exposure, he agreed to move his family from Florida to Washington, DC, to take a full-time job at Walter Reed.

One of the many indoctrination courses at Walter Reed was the required "dreaded" information course on hospitality. The Disney executive was a key speaker. His lecture on how to create a hospitable environment was extraordinary. As a result, I went right back to my private office to change the way it was set up. I got rid of a lot of clutter, which is a distraction to patients. Courtesy and graciousness make a difference in an environment whether large or small.

The Disney executive illustrated a major point about hospitality by asking the audience what was the most frequently asked question at Disney World. The answer, "What time is the three o'clock parade?" The three o'clock parade in Disney World occurs at various times depending on where you are standing when the parade passes you by. It might be three thirty; it might be three forty-five. His point: There are no stupid questions.

His work and that of others shows in the results. Almost everyone at Walter Reed greets and speaks to one another. The cafeteria is crowded and sometimes mobbed. Throughout are many soldiers in wheelchairs, some with two or three limbs missing. It is a sobering sight, and yet they all look like they're managing well. Modern surgery produces many effective artificial limbs and appendages. I learned, however, that physical trauma is one thing and psychic trauma is another.

After I completed an extensive number of indoctrination and credentialing courses, I was scheduled to see my first soldier. While I was scheduled to do the interview over closed circuit telepsychiatry, a medium unfamiliar to me, I noticed in myself an unusual degree of apprehension. Checking with colleagues, they confirmed a similar reaction. It wasn't just the technology or the complexity of the electronic medical records. It was also the enormity of the task. I knew these soldiers suffered, yet I had no idea of the complexity of their past and present lives. The first soldier was beyond my expectations.

He was very depressed both chronically and acutely. He had a suicide plan, which I confirmed was plausible and possible. I proposed three options for working on this problem. I suggested he could make a choice of which plan we would work on. Frustrated, he picked up a trashcan and threw it at me and walked out of the room. The hundreds of miles between us insulated me from the flying trashcan but created a logistical problem in how to save him from himself. Fortunately, the Army's enlightened suicidal prevention program allowed me to contact personnel on his base to help me with the situation.

A few days later came a soldier brandishing a knife. A routine question in the waiting room, "Where does your spouse live?" prompted the response, "If you find out, let me know." As the soldier pulled the knife and walked into the viewing room, I began receiving telephone calls saying that security had surrounded the booth and was prepared to arrest him following my interview. All of this and I had not even seen the soldier.

Needless to say, I felt obligated to ask him about his plans and he responded by giving me a detailed description of how he intended to kill his wife and do it in a way that would make her suffer in the most extreme manner. This soldier has suffered though his multiple deployments and now was going to make his wife suffer for the pains that he believed she was causing him. I knew immediately that he was going to test all that I had learned in forty years of practicing psychiatry.

We spent an hour talking about a variety of issues. He explained the necessity of carrying the knife. He couldn't sleep, and he had a hard time eating because he had no appetite. He couldn't shop for groceries because he couldn't be in crowds. The knife was necessary in case somebody bumped him.

He had tried alcohol to numb his psychic pain. Beating up a policeman, an arrest, and a long hospitalization helped him realize alcohol was not the solution. He was denied admission to an anger management course because he so frightened the intake worker.

She determined that the other members in the course would be too intimidated by his comments.

By the end of the hour, I decided to tell him simply that his plan to kill his wife was not a good idea. I explained that no matter how angry he was with her, it was not a good way to treat people and it could create a lot of trouble for him. I further explained that he simply couldn't come back with a knife because it makes people too upset. Although he protested about his need for self-defense, he understood how the presence of the knife might be upsetting to others. He agreed to return to discuss how to more effectively deal with the real problems his wife was presenting. I have no doubt that the course on hospitality was a part of my response. No one should treat or be treated this way.

I explained to the soldier that if he could agree to come back and work on these problems, I would call his base and tell the security police outside of the video booth that he should be free to go. He agreed, and he returned for months to work on these matters. He decided that he could not be an effective soldier and could not be deployed in a combat zone and therefore should leave the Army. He has come a long way in dealing with his trauma, but adjustment in civilian life will be complicated.

These evaluations are multifaceted. In one hour, the soldier is introduced to video conferencing, a history is taken, a plan is formulated, medications and psychotherapy are discussed, and an electronic medical record of this discussion is made. When the soldier plans to commit suicide or kill one of his commanders, it is difficult to "pull it all together" in one hour. An entire systemic plan needs to be in place. After a while, PTSD can become infectious. Listening to and dealing with the accumulated trauma of one or many soldiers can be traumatizing to the person listening. No wonder soldiers often find others only superficially interested in their problems. Many say that they can only talk to someone who really understands what happened.

This accumulated trauma creates traumatized relationships with their intimate others. How do spouses, separated for months, often caring for their mutual children, find the strength and resolve to be supportive and understanding? Some soldiers awaken by noises in the middle of the night and misidentify a sleeping spouse as an enemy. More commonly, nightmares lead to flailing in bed at whoever is nearby.

One of the most difficult listening problems I had is the following story. A soldier related that he and two or three of his colleagues were on patrol. Suddenly, the others were "vaporized" by an explosion. After dealing with this emergency, he and others were left to collect body parts into bags. He complained of nightmares about this experience seven nights a week, week after week. It is difficult to know what to say. "Thank you for your service" seems inadequate. I listened.

Frankly, I dreaded his return. He was absent a long time. When he did return, I asked him how he was. He reported that he had just returned from visiting his mother and father. His mother was dying from metastatic breast cancer and he had spent two weeks with them while she was in hospice. He noted that he had never seen a death from natural causes. He found the hospice experience very comforting. He was helpful to both parents and gained great comfort from them in return. He said the nightmares were going away. Upon further questioning, he said that being part of a natural dying process helped him put his war experience in a different perspective. Much later, after a long vacation with his surviving father, he again reported how helpful he thought the experience had been in discussing denial, anger, and grief with his father. The nightmares? They were gone! I learned that not many twentysomethings have had much experience with death as a natural process.

One can read more about these experiences in the book *War* by Sebastian Junger, author of the *Perfect Storm*, or see the movie *Restrepo*, based on his book. The intensity of prolonged conflict leaves many to fear the "silence of American civilian life." The adaptation to "normal life" is difficult, and many long to return to battle.

Although soldiers do fight for each other as much as anything, they also speak of the addiction to battle. Junger's book demonstrates, and soldiers confirm, that the adrenaline "high" of intense combat is better than a cocaine high and lasts longer. The author ably notes the biological and evolutionary roots of this addiction supported by society and amply reinforced by "older men," past their prime, making decisions to send younger men into proxy battles.

Although many point out the apparent futility of the current strategy of this war, both of these wars, and the current and future effect they will have on our society, is a far more complex problem. George Will argues in his article "The Second-most Dangerous American" that so far "we probably have paid no more than 20 percent of the eventual costs" of the war.

We need to ask ourselves what will hundreds of young men addicted to fighting do when they return to "normal" society. Some describe the irony of their inability to participate in a simple July Fourth Independence Day celebration because exploding firecrackers startle them into battle. We also need to ask ourselves whether our society has an addiction to war as a way of dealing with conflict with others who are viewed as different or threatening our way of life. Is there a tendency to send young men and women off to battle to heroically defend "our way" of life? Junger's book and the movies are good places to begin thinking about these issues. I hope these essays will offer a similar opportunity to remember these young men and women caught in a maelstrom beyond their wildest expectations. We need to pray for them daily.

On one of my first days working at Walter Reed Army Medical Center, I was standing by myself waiting for the elevator. Out of the corner of my eye I noticed an approaching wheelchair. As I turned, I could see the oncoming soldier had no arms or legs. A stub of an elbow operated the steering mechanism. Before I could catch my breath to say anything, the empty elevator arrived. "After you, sir," he said. Speechless, I followed his suggestion. In a nutshell, this episode captures part of what our wars create. Confrontation with unspeakable trauma! What are we to do? I learned that saying something "unthinkable in polite society" like, "How did you lose your arms and legs?" can really reduce the tension.

This experience introduced me to physical trauma but did not prepare me for my first patient. Little did I appreciate that I would soon be dealing not only with physical trauma but the experience of killing. Killing the enemy is the bottom line of what our wars have been all about. Those armies that determine best how to kill most of the enemy are more likely to be successful. In the American Civil War, the North triumphed over the South in part because the former had more soldiers to fight and die than the latter.

On a personal level, killing can be one of the most intimate acts a human can experience. The more empathic one is the more difficult killing can be. The more asocial one is the easier killing can be. The more a soldier can dehumanize an enemy the easier to kill him.

On a societal level, moral clarity of leadership is critical in killing. Presumably, the more clear the purpose of war the easier the personal killing and its psychological aftermath and residue. President Lincoln, a most empathic person, decided that Grant and Sherman were the generals who could win the Civil War. They agreed that the enemy army had to be destroyed in order to win the war.

Recent studies suggest that 750,000 Americans died in that war, a number equivalent to 7.5 million citizens in today's population. The unprecedented American killing was undertaken and accomplished in part because of the moral clarity of its purpose. Lincoln determined to first save the Union and later to free the slaves. Despite the overwhelming carnage, most everyone would agree on the nobility of these goals. Today, citizens want the goals of a war accomplished but want to avoid being the person killed.

The moral clarity of leadership makes personal killing easier. The psychological residue of killing is soothed by the clarity of purpose.

Society absorbs the psychological residues of death and personal trauma the more closely knit its citizens. Individual grief can be absorbed by collective grief.

The world watched 9/11 bring these issues into sharp focus. Watching innocent victims jump from burning buildings cannot help but stir emotional responses from the observer. Three thousand Americans killed in one day. Our society demanded a response. It was probably impossible for our political leadership to respond in any other manner than we did. The enemy seemed clear. We thought we knew whom to kill.

We declared a war on terrorism. See Callimachi's February 2018 report in *The New York Times* about the political leadership response that led to strategic wars in Afghanistan and later Iraq. As in Vietnam, there were multiple tactical victories in both Afghanistan and Iraq. Our forces designed for short decisive campaigns on a large scale are effective at killing and dominating. Once the response to our invasion and the insurgencies develop, our Army is not so effective. Counterinsurgency—setting up governments that endure and protect its population—has not been our strength. Defining the enemy and knowing who to kill defines the war. Once the enemy can be everyone, our moral compass is unclear and our goals are elusive. We are now contemplating unending war with a less than clear purpose. Even the military leadership agrees more civilian input into our war policy is required.

These deaths and injuries between 9/11 and now, with the possible exception of Osama bin Laden's assassination, are morally questionable as Fallows stated in his article in *The Atlantic,* January/ February 2015. By 2017, the only morally agreed upon reaction was the killing of bin Laden, the architect of 9/11. The war in Afghanistan continues with over 3,500 soldiers killed and 111,000 Afghans killed. The war in Iraq with fewer Americans now that in the past continues with 4,500 soldiers killed, over 30,000 injured, and at least 100,000 Iraqis dead. The war in Syria continues. There is an ongoing democracy in Iraq, but at what price? Knowing in advance the future human toil, would Iraqi citizens have voted for democracy?

Is the American public prepared to write a blank check to engage in wars for which we are unprepared? The answers to these questions are not clear. What is clear is that the American public appears willing to allow the military to engage in these wars as long as someone else is going to fight them. Once assigned the task of fighting, the military appears willing to continue the wars while asking for more time and money.

The public is eager to thank our soldiers for their service, but we do not really know what to do with them. It appears that our civilian leaders share our dilemma. Thomas Brennan (2017) in his latest book, *Shooting Ghosts,* says, "People love to tell me I look fine. My wounds are invisible to most people but visible to me. War wounded my soul." If the public does not take our soldiers seriously, the public will not take our military seriously. The military, untended by civilian oversight, will suffer. The American public is not willing to make the tough decisions as long as the alternative allows someone else to suffer.

Adm. Mike Mullen, the former chairman of the Joint Chiefs of Staff says, "It's become just too easy to go to war" (Fallows, 2015). The admiral thinks the American public and the military need to reengage, and become more involved, with each other. He believes that by shrinking the size of the Army now, the next time we consider war, the American people will have to agree and do so by putting more skin in the game. More civilians will have to join the service in order to carry on the war and be "inconvenienced." He believes that the country has suffered from lack of public involvement in the military. I believe the servicemen and servicewomen carry our suffering and grief, and we owe it to them to listen to make their grief a collective grief.

I decided to do that, to listen to soldiers in 2010. Here in these next essays are stories that I heard. The first four essays are about killing. Killing the enemy is critical to winning war. The military trains soldiers to distinguish between necessary killing and murder. Rules of engagement are important. Unfortunately, in the cauldron of battle, it is not always easy to make distinctions. And soldiers experience emotional fallout. These essays focus on killing anonymous enemies, spouses, teenagers, and themselves by suicide.

# PART I

# KILLING

CHAPTER ONE

# KILLING SPOUSES

### *"If You Know My Wife's Location, Let me Know"*

"Doc, next time is the last time I will meet with you. I am getting out of the Army."

"So soon?" I asked.

"I have really given you an education," he added.

Yes, he had.

In 2010, he was one of the first service members I had seen. Before I turned on the closed circuit television, I received a call from his remote location. "We have surrounded the room with security police and are ready to arrest him as soon as you are finished," said the caller. I, of course, not having spoken to the soldier, had no idea what was going on.

He arrived in the waiting room brandishing a knife. Working on the pre-visit questionnaire, he responded about his wife's location by announcing that if they found her they should let him know. Apparently, it took them little time to conclude that he was planning to kill his wife. Regardless of his chief complaint, his immediate concern was the impending arrest.

I began by asking him how this situation had arisen. He had returned from his second deployment and had obviously suffered a lot of trauma. He said he needed the knife for protection. Sometimes in crowds he was bumped. The knife was for defense.

"What is the story with you and your wife?" I asked.

"She has made me suffer, and now I want to make her suffer. I am going to kill her as slowly as possible beginning by cutting off her fingers one by one. When I have finished with them, I am going to cut off her toes. I know how to prolong it."

He seemed serious, and I knew I had my work cut out for me. I realized I would have to rely on everything I had learned in the last forty years in psychiatry to deal with this problem. The easy solution was to have him arrested. He would go to jail for making threats, and the problem before me would disappear. I was tempted. But that was not why I took this job and not what I wanted to do. In spite of the threats, there was something very appealing about this man. Underneath this bravado was a very frightened person.

We spent an hour talking about how he had arrived at this point in his life. He had been hospitalized for a month after he beat up a policeman. He had been in alcohol rehabilitation and was now on probation. He was refused admission to an anger management program because he so frightened the intake worker. She thought no one in the group could tolerate the intensity of his anger. After listening for an hour, I put aside all my training as I thought common sense should prevail. I told him that killing his wife was simply not a good idea. He would create a lot of trouble for himself. Besides, no matter how badly she might have treated him, she did not deserve to die. Also, he could not bring the knife back because he scared everybody. To my surprise and without too much protest, he agreed. He has attended sessions weekly for the past two plus years.

Today, he says, "I have a rather demented and dark side to myself. I can be sick and heartless and even have the recipe for the perfect crime. I know about torture, control, proper location, and disposal of the victim. I have learned that if I am sufficiently isolated, without structure I can become comfortable with criminal behavior."

For a long time, he needed serious medication to keep these ideas in check. His irritability, hyperalertness, and anger were such that firecracker explosions on the Fourth of July did him in. A returning soldier unable to celebrate our nation's most patriotic holiday!

He has worked hard. Sobriety, anger management class, raising his own pets, and even a reasonable divorce have helped. He found the personal resources to obtain a paternity determination on his wife's child. Proving it was not his child relieved him of all those stressful child custody payments. The judge would not order back to him these prior unjustified payments, but the service member had made his point about undeserved suffering. His wife had been making him pay child support for a child she conceived while he was deployed.

He has a better perspective on his life: his divorce, his parents' divorce, the long time in an orphanage, the recent death of a beloved grandmother, his deployments. Medically disabled, he will receive disability payments, money for college, and even possibly Social Security. "I served my country, and I deserve it," he says.

"My goal now is keeping myself off the six o'clock news," he says, chuckling. "As long as my name is not there, I have had a good day. I used to be in left field and although I may not have made it to 'the right field,' I am well on my way." Pretty good thinking for a guy who perhaps might have been a wife killer!

And yes, he is right about another thing: He did teach me a lot.

I don't know if he, as a potential wife killer, is one of many. I do know that as a service member suffering with PTSD, he is one of the many. Killing others, being the subject of enemy rockets and improvised explosive devices (IEDs), even being associated with combat contributes to PTSD. These men see, hear, feel, and speak of death. Sometimes, they kill others and sometimes themselves. He has not made his six o'clock news, but far too many others have made our six o'clock news.

What can we as a society do to change this news? Talking about how we send these men off to do "our work" is a beginning. Talking directly to soldiers about their trauma and PTSD symptoms—their story—clearly helps. So does medication. What is it that will help heal these scars in our society? Do you want your son or daughter or grandchildren to follow in their footsteps?

## PROFESSIONAL REFLECTIONS

My problem was how to address a clearly dangerous situation. I was located at Walter Reed Department of Psychiatry, Washington, DC, and the soldier was at Fort Hood, Texas. Everyone at Fort Hood—the nurse, the patient, the military police—were quite anxious. Was their anxiety and concern appropriate to the threat posed by this soldier?

This clinic was the same as the one in which Army psychiatrist Maj. Nidal Hassan, on November 5, 2009, had murdered fourteen people and wounded twenty-nine. Hassan, a US Army psychiatrist, was an American-born Muslim of Palestinian descent. He received his psychiatric training at Walter Reed Department of Psychiatry in the same building in which I was sitting. These murders in the Texas clinic must be contributing to their anxiety. The killings would influence the way the clinical staff was assessing the threat posed by this soldier.

Anxiety can be infectious. It spreads in concentric circles like the wave of water after a stone is dropped in a pond. It proceeds outward from the hole in the water made by the stone, in this case the patient. The anxiety jumps to the next circle, the family, and the next circle, society. Unless interrupted, the anxiety just reverberates back and forth between circles.

Their staff knew I worked with people who worked with the killer, no doubt enhancing their anxiety. I saw no way to address that problem directly, but I knew it must be contributing to this situation.

There are two ways to deal with this acute problem presented by the soldier. I could invoke the assistance of the military police, one of the outer layers of the circle to contain the situation. That action would contain the anxiety but not deal with the needs of this soldier, who despite his threats came for help. Or I could turn to him, the source of the current anxiety, and stand in the way of these reverberating emotional circuits. I could try to tamp down this shockwave that he was generating. I chose the latter knowing my colleagues would probably favor the former, i.e., be on the safe side.

That day, I knew the bulwark had to be me. I was tempted to just call the police, but that was not why I took this job and not what I wanted to do. Despite the threats, there was something very appealing about this man. Underneath his bravado was a very frightened person.

I decided to start at the beginning and ask him how this situation had arisen. He recounted his deployments. The constant stress contributed to his hypervigilance. He was alert to the enemy everywhere, hence his need to carry a knife. Constant threats in battle numb one's capacity for empathy. People everywhere are seen as the enemy. Alcohol does not work long term. Anger management classes can help, but he was too frightening.

This soldier was losing his ability to distinguish between the battlefield and the safety of home. The Army calls it Battle Mind. It is just how one perceives the environment. I knew there was no point in arguing with him. Saying, "Hey, buddy, you really are safe," would not work. That is clearly not how he felt. Not only could he not distinguish the battlefield from the home front, but neither could he tell friend from foe. Somehow, he had identified his wife as the enemy and he was going to torture and murder her.

I wanted to get to know soldiers, and I hoped a good relationship with him would be helpful. Despite these very sadistic threats, I do not know why, but I liked him. I had to be cautious as he could have been just a sociopath who was enticing me to take a risk with his threats.

He needed a different frame of reference, not Battle Mind, but common sense. His plans to kill his wife—whatever perceived wrong that might avenge—were not tactically smart and would land him in jail. Besides, he needed to remain a human being and she did also. Whatever her perceived sin, she did not deserve what he was planning.

I was surprised and pleased that he agreed to abide by the common sense plan. I knew my colleagues might not agree with my action. After all, the Tarasoff decision required mental health workers to warn third parties who were in danger. Did I have to find his wife and tell her of his plans?

We met weekly for two years. Gradually, the issues that led to his plans emerged. He has a very dark side that requires outside structure to keep him intact. He needs personal and social structure, even a dog to comfort him. He used the court system "to fight" his wife and did so successfully. His humor, keeping "myself off the six o'clock news," helped.

Not every soldier in this situation keeps himself off the six o'clock news. There are returning veterans, however, who will make the six o'clock news. A solid common sense relationship with each veteran helps. Can you find a way to be one of those relationships? It does not have to be with a soldier as troubled as this one. It can just be with someone who served for you.

CHAPTER TWO

# KILLING ENEMIES

## *"Maybe He Was Just Looking for a Television"*

"Teenager? Terrorist? Or both?" Those were the questions the convoy leader in Afghanistan kept asking himself. Almost ten years ago, a teenager jumped into the front seat of his vehicle, startling him and requiring him to make a split-second response, the result of which would last both their lifetimes. One died and one lived.

Now, as this soldier's own son reaches the same age as the teenager who faced him in the jeep that day, the soldier sits and tells his story for the first time. After multiple deployments on three continents, he "knew" the enemy could be anyone anywhere. As the commander of the convoy, he had to be vigilant. Service in Somalia had taught him that one never knows who the enemy is. That day in question, his convoy was surrounded by civilians. His driver was not adequately protecting their vehicle from the crowds. Tensions were high. "Kids" seemed to be everywhere. Were they just "kids," or were they trained as the enemy? Whatever the answer, the soldier and the teenager faced each other, each speaking a different language.

The soldier explains that as a teenager himself, he had been an excellent student, straight A's. A three-sport athlete, he received a full athletic college scholarship. Only an injury kept him from an athletic career. A career in the military has been a satisfactory and successful substitute. Yet, now after further injury, he was unable to make a final deployment with his unit. Separated from his buddies, he began to feel guilty about "not being there." And the guilt got him thinking.

His marriage has gone well. He and his wife have two healthy children. Who knew his worry about his son's continued health would be a factor in his "chief complaint"? He has suppressed that fateful day in Afghanistan for almost ten years. The experience is not something he would discuss with his wife. Too traumatic for her! But now that his older son is the same age as the teenager who had startled him by jumping into his vehicle that fateful day, it is always on his mind. At some level, the soldier knows that his current overly protective behavior toward his teenage son would not bring life back to the Afghan teen. Yet, similar age, combined with guilt, has become a fateful juxtaposition!

His current guilt about being separated from his buddies also triggers memories of the prior unresolved guilt of that fateful day. Nightmares, irritability, depression, chronic physical pain, and concern for the welfare of his son are now all part of his story. Although he believes he made the right decision to protect himself and his unit, he knows he remains troubled.

He is a religious person, goes to church regularly, and thinks that God understands. He is not certain his wife would. Their son wants to go to the Air Force Academy. If his wife knew of this soldier's fateful day, would she prevent their son from entering military service?

He has not discussed it with his chaplain. Was it really a decision or a reaction? Was it just the wrong place at the wrong time? Did he experience bad "moral luck"? Was he responsible but not culpable? Did he and the teenager both play a part?

These are questions that have been—surprisingly—seldom addressed in any systematic way by society. In a 2017 article in *The New Yorker* magazine, "The Sorrow and the Shame of the Accidental Killer," Alice Gregory addresses them. She says there are no self-help books for accidentally killing another person—"no therapeutic protocols, publically listed support groups, or therapists who specialize in their treatment."

Gregory's article further states that the Centers for Disease Control and Prevention "lists nearly one hundred and forty-seven thousand unintentional injury deaths" in 2015. Neither the Insurance Institute for Highway Safety nor the National Transportation Safety Board track people who unintentionally cause the death of another. Gregory further writes that neither the American Counseling Association, the American Psychological Association, nor the American Automobile Association know of any experts in this field.

Maybe no one pays any attention to the perpetrators of accidental killings because they are such incredibly random events. Yet, no matter how random the event, the reaction and response is not. In the film *Manchester by the Sea* (2016), a young father accidentally causes a house fire that kills his three children. The accidental fire leads the parents, in their grief, to divorce. One of the most poignant scenes in film history occurs as they meet years later, trying to explain to each other what happened to their marriage. Grief ripped it apart. They were overwhelmed by the enormity of it all.

Gregory brings up the problem of "moral luck," an issue that has been addressed by philosophers from Aristotle to Kant to Bernard Williams (1981) and Thomas Nagel (1976). Gregory noted that "Jeff McMahan, a professor of moral philosophy at Oxford, says . . . 'People who are not culpable can nevertheless be responsible.' "

And what are these people, these accidental killers, to do? Gregory notes that Maimonides, the Jewish philosopher, argues "that in the collective grief the individual grief is assuaged." The ritual of shared conversation is critical.

As I listened further to this soldier, I knew what he needed to do and said, "You must discuss this situation with your wife." He did. It took months of work individually and together. The receptive social system or, in his case, his nuclear and extended family, is a resource for "mending a broken heart." Some grief is so monumental that it cannot be contained within an individual or within a relationship but must become collective.

The patient reports a 75-80 percent improvement in his symptoms. He no longer views his son as his soldier. The days of not being able to get out of bed are gone. He claims a 95 percent improvement in his home life.

He still wonders, *What if that kid who jumped into my vehicle and whom I killed was just curious about the television computer screen on the dashboard of my vehicle?*

[i] *Williams, Bernard (1981). "Moral Luck." Moral Luck: Philosophical Papers 1973-1980. Cambridge: Cambridge University Press. pp. 20–39. OCLC 7597880.*

[ii] *Nagel, Thomas (1979). "Moral Luck" (PDF). Mortal Questions. Cambridge: Cambridge University Press. pp. 24–38. OCLC 4135927.*

## PROFESSIONAL REFLECTION

As this soldier told his story, I could see tragedy written all over his face—the pain of not knowing for certain, yet, at some level knowing for certain, he had made a mistake in judgment. But was it a decision or just a reaction? Could he be held accountable for a split-second action in the fog of war? Hindsight plays tricks on the mind, suggesting now ten years later that he possessed the luxury of reflection before acting.

The accidental death of the teenager, a casualty of war, is a real tragedy. And I had an obligation to help him find his way out of this dark hole. I have no experience in knowing what to say or do in this situation. Aristotle's

*Poetics* suggests a truly tragic figure must be the average person who by his actions ends up in misery. This poor soldier qualifies. Nightmares, irritability, depression, chronic physical pain, and concern for the welfare of his son are now all part of his miserable story. Medication can remedy all these symptoms. But that is not his problem.

His problem is that he killed an innocent teenager, someone else's son, who was curious and maybe impulsive but certainly not, in hindsight, an enemy. Aristotle suggests that real tragedy must contain a horrible or evil deed. The deed must be more than killing the enemy or peripheral person but rather a family member. Killing someone else's family member is close enough to Aristotle's definition to qualify this soldier as a tragic figure.

This soldier survived ten years with few problems by compartmentalizing these issues. He did not talk with his wife, his chaplain, or his physician. If he kept them from the pain, he could keep himself from the pain.

Life continues. As the future evolves, one discovers present day reminders of the past. His unit from which he received so much emotional support deployed without him. Current guilt about being separated from his buddies triggered memories of the prior unresolved guilt of that fateful day.

I could tell him that the Centers for Disease Control and Prevention says nearly 147,000 unintentional deaths occurred in a recent year. Hardly reassuring. I could tell him that there are no experts in helping someone who unintentionally committed a horrible deed.

I know he would hear those comments as my pulling away from him. I know he does not need this type of emotional distancing from a caretaker. He needs to be surrounded by and cared for by those people he cares for, his family. I took a chance. I did not know. I only hoped his family would be receptive. They were. It took months of work individually and together. The receptive social system or, in his case, his nuclear and extended family, is a resource for "mending a broken heart." Some grief is so monumental that it cannot be contained within an individual or within a relationship but must become collective.

America has compartmentalized this tragedy by assigning it to the 1 percent of our population who are engaged. The other 99 percent of us have it so compartmentalized and are so emotionally distant from the killing that we do not even think about it, let alone speak of it. Seeing the faces of the dead on nightly television is as close as we get. And at what price? Are we no longer together in service of our country?

Just as I felt with this soldier, we have no experience in knowing what to say or do in this situation. Where does our path lie? We are involved in the making of a tragedy of continuous war. We are decent people who collectively have allowed horrible deeds to happen, no matter whether intentionally or out of our ignorance. We are the wealthiest group in the world and also among the least happy. Aristotle says a true tragic hero must be in misery. We are there.

But our collective path must lead us beyond our own tribe to all Americans. Our conversations need not lead to universal military service, but they should lead to national service. I suspect that we do not want to confront our responsibilities and the associated grief. Beginning a conversation with soldiers is a good first step. I suspect we will find them to be great teachers about tragedy.

# CHAPTER THREE

# KILLING ENEMIES AND KILLING OURSELVES

## *"Living With Death—It's Just Their Job"*

A forty-year-old first sergeant left a message canceling her appointment. The staff sergeant in her Special Ops unit had committed suicide. Her message sat in the back of my mind for the next twenty-four hours. Finally, I called her back, leaving this message:

> *"I was sorry to hear about the death of the staff sergeant in your unit. I assume he worked with or for you. I assume you have contacted a number of your colleagues and have been talking with them. From my experience I think it is important to talk about suicide—for yourself first of all and for your soldiers as individuals and as members of your unit—especially for the future functioning of the unit. If you wish to talk about the effects of this suicide on yourself and others—or talk just about death—please call me back."*

Her return call came within the hour.

The first sergeant said she was fine, that she appreciated the call. Yet, with little prodding, she accepted an emergency appointment. She gave me the facts: The staff sergeant worked for her; she knew him and his wife well. They both were in the military and had just decided to retire. They had civilian jobs and were planning to move within the next few months. He seemed fine with no sign of distress. The first sergeant had no idea why he shot himself, especially having a wife and two small children.

It was not long before she acknowledged that this was the third suicide in her unit in the past few months and that a few years ago her mother had committed suicide. *Where to begin?* I thought.

"What type of work does your Special Ops unit do?" I asked.

"We monitor television screens all day."

"And what do you see?" I asked.

"We are looking at targets."

"Human targets?" I asked. "Is the purpose of this monitoring to kill people?" I wondered out loud.

"Yes," she said, but she added, "We are very careful to recognize a person's gait, movements, and various individual features. We have cameras on the ground, showing guys kicking down doors, and also aerial cameras. We know who we are killing. We work in twelve-hour shifts and are debriefed after each shift. A behavioral health specialist is available for consultation if the work is too stressful."

Trying to get my mind around how stressful this activity must be, I asked, "How often do you kill people—once a month, once a week, once a day?"

"Every day," she said. Sensing my disbelief, she offered, "It is not a job for everybody. My husband thinks it's terrible. Some people see it like a video game. Others do not have the stomach for it."

I suggested that three suicides in the past few months in this relatively small unit sounded like stress to me. She acknowledged how important it was for her to be available to everyone in the unit to talk about the suicide and to have a proper funeral. So, when I asked about the soldier's wife and children, she said that his wife had taken the children and "gone home." No official contact had been made between the wife's unit and the husband's unit. She explained that there was no official mechanism to have contact between units about these matters.

I cannot stop thinking about the military unit—just as I think about *family*—even though the military unit is not my patient. It is important for the members of the unit to talk about and "to metabolize" a trauma. The soldiers who worked with and for this staff sergeant should be talking to his wife, just as family members should reach out to one another. My patient agreed. She said she would be attending the funeral and would see what could be done.

As weeks passed, everything "returned back to normal." The military had a proper funeral; the wife and family did not attend. No one spoke with the soldier's wife, and no one knows if there was a separate family funeral. Where was he buried? Arlington? What type of real or symbolic closure is there for his widow and children, for this military unit, or for our society?

The spirit of the Army is built on altruism and caring for others. Does the service member/widow think her husband gave his life for the unit and his country? Or does she think the Army (job) killed her husband? Does she wonder where his colleagues and their altruism are now?

My patient and these soldiers in her unit are back at work monitoring television sets and killing human targets. Is that what they are going to do with the rest of *their* lives? Does their altruism exclude his widow and his children once that soldier whom they had worked beside has fallen? Do they even think about it? Have they fully done their job?

The war in Iraq is over for the United States except for Special Ops. The war in Afghanistan is over for the United States except for Special Ops. The war in Syria never started for the United States except for Special Ops. None of these wars ever began for 99 percent of non-military American people.

I am surprised to learn that "our side" is killing people every day. Some of us who are killing them are then killing ourselves in response! Most of us are on the sidelines, and we are not watching. We are as disconnected from the killing as these soldiers apparently are disconnected from the widow and her children. Are we willfully blind, or is the killing just part of the background noise that we have become accustomed to in our everyday living?

## PROFESSIONAL REFLECTIONS

How we kill the enemy has changed. In past wars, the killing was more up close and personal. Hand-to-hand combat defined much of war. Certainly that type of killing persists today. Rifles, then automatic weapons, cannons, bombs, and nuclear warheads all make killing more scientific and sophisticated. We now have highly specific ways of following and killing targets remotely. We can kill enemies from halfway around the world with a touch of a button. Targeted remote killing of high-value suspects may be more moral, producing less collateral damage.

As I listened to this soldier's story, I thought that I could not be hearing what I knew I was hearing. I asked very simple questions to make certain I got the facts straight. Daily, remote, televised, watched on monitors high-value targeted killing in twelve-hour shifts. Regular mental health debriefings determine if you "have the stomach for the work"!

Targeted killings must address two basic questions: 1) Is the target definitely the enemy? and 2) Will attacking the target harm civilians? Apparently, despite this precise air campaign, we have killed 3,000 innocent civilians in Iraq alone (Khan, 2017).

Of the more than 27,500 strikes in Iraq and Syria, the military admits to a mistake 1/157 times. *The New York Times* estimates a mistake 1/5 times. Despite this difference of opinion, one has to be impressed with the surgical precision of the killings. But also, one has to be impressed with the fallout—the number of soldiers who are killing themselves after they anonymously kill targets.

What is going on here? I ask myself.

There is no official mechanism for the dead soldier's peers to speak with his widowed wife. Is his suicide just a message from the dead, saying, "I was not okay with what I was doing but could not talk about it?"

Do the innocent civilians feel their "hearts and minds" are being converted by these precise killings?

This shift work, scheduled killings, is another form of compartmentalizing the job of war. Yet, even as the nature of killing changes, apparently, the grief remains—for the individual, the unit, the family, and maybe for society at large? In Burns and Novick's documentary film series, *The Vietnam War,* an interview with an enemy soldier produced the following quote: "War does not determine who is right, only who is left." And who is bereft? Within our soldiers lies the residue of our collective grief. We and they need to share it.

# CHAPTER FOUR
# SUICIDE

## *"I Looked But Did Not See It Coming"*

Rarely does a soldier enter my office and become so profoundly sad and upset that it is difficult to find out what happened. Such was the case with this thirty-eight-year-old noncommissioned female officer who arrived recently. All she could say between crying spells was, "He did not show up for work."

"Who?" I asked.

She described an outstanding soldier with whom she had been deployed to Iraq. Although an enlisted soldier, he was the unspoken leader of the unit. He volunteered to take photos of individual soldiers, write stories of their experiences, and send them to their families. He kept up the spirits of soldiers and their families. Everyone in the unit went to him for guidance. When the unit completed its tour of duty and returned to the United States, the soldier was also completing the terms of his service and was being discharged. He had a high IQ, good social skills, and scored well on aptitude tests. He was enrolled in college and had a bright future at age twenty-two.

Transitioning out of the military can be difficult. One of this officer's jobs was to conduct an exit interview. She was in charge of the base suicide prevention program so she knew what to look for and what questions to ask. She had received all the training. She taught others what to monitor. She knew the "key words and signs" to observe. To her ear, the soldier sounded healthy and ready to leave. He had family, was connected to fellow soldiers, and not depressed. He was *not* impulsive, always well-groomed and well-behaved with no behavioral health problems. He was a leader. Yet, it is never possible to know what is on another's mind.

When he did not show up for work, she went to his room. "It smelled of death," she said. "There he was hanging from the ceiling. Apparently, I missed something." As she spoke, I could see the pain in her face and her posture as if she were still looking at the dead soldier hanging from the ceiling. His peers apparently kept secret that every weekend he would drink alcohol to the point of unconsciousness. Is binge drinking by young people so commonplace that no one thought it was worth mentioning? How could she not have been made aware of this fact?

Her description of what she observed felt to me that it had happened yesterday, but actually it was one year ago. Why after a year of suffering could she not forgive herself? So, I asked, "Do you blame yourself for the loss of this soldier?"

"Since childhood, every time I got close to people, I feared losing them and then the funeral experience made it so much more complicated."

She and four other soldiers accompanied his casket to the family funeral. Upon introducing herself and offering condolences to his parents, the soldier's mother turned to her and said, "It is your fault. I put my son in your care, and you allowed him to kill himself." Not only had she been blaming herself, but now the blame came from outside as well. It is never possible to know what is on another's mind.

I wondered with whom she had talked to share her guilt and her perceived responsibility. "Not with my husband," she said, although he was also in the military. "His baggage from deployments is worse than mine," she said. "Not with my peers, either" she said. "We are expected to keep busy and keep going. Keeping busy works for a while. The military spends millions for suicide prevention and counseling, and yet there are no programs for leaders whose soldiers have killed themselves like my soldier did."

Our time was over and yet I knew virtually nothing about this patient's background—an essential for a proper evaluation. I wondered what was really on her mind behind all that pain. As she exited my office, I realized that I faced the same dilemma as did she when that soldier was leaving her unit. I asked her if, being so distressed, she had ever thought of hurting herself. "I love myself and my family. I would never hurt my family by hurting myself." A strong enough response for me! I thought it was all right for her to leave. The reasons behind her intense feelings of responsibility would have to wait until the next visit.

Most soldiers are indoctrinated with banding together to care for fellow soldiers, but her reaction over the loss seemed excessive. On the next visit, I asked how she accounted for such strong feelings of responsibility for the death of this soldier. She said she had done virtually everything possible to prevent it. She acknowledged being called "Mother Teresa" by her family since childhood. And yes, her childhood history revealed many clues about what I called "ambiguous" deaths and her sense of responsibility for ones that were hard to explain like the death of this soldier.

This female noncommissioned officer's feelings of responsibility probably stemmed from the early loss of her father, for which she inexplicably blamed herself. This emotional reaction was cemented by other family deaths. Her older adolescent sister died in bed. She was the one who found her. Her adult brother died mysteriously. Her firstborn son died after ten days of life. If one survives all these experiences with a self-blaming response, it is almost a prescription for becoming a "caretaker" as an adult.

Is this the type of soldier typically drawn to the military? One who cares so much for others' lives that it becomes a total personal burden? The Army teaches defense of country by banding together, by killing the enemy and protecting others, and by what some might call *altruism*. This teaching may be effective in *preventing* deaths, but what happens when some deaths *do* occur?

When a soldier dies in combat, fellow soldiers are troubled and feel guilty about not having been able to save that comrade. When a soldier kills himself in his own room, fellow soldiers may be even more troubled about not saving their comrade. The Army can teach altruism, which is critical for the survival of the unit. But when that altruism—that concern for others—is built on top of her type of family structure, it can stretch human empathy to an unhealthy vulnerability.

At this moment, in the face of this death, *forgiveness,* not altruism, is sorely needed. One can never fully know what is in another's mind. For this service member to forgive herself for all she believes she "missed," she first needs to *recognize* that forgiveness is involved here. Forgiveness does not seem to have entered her mind. I hope that I can help her find a place in her own mind for self-forgiveness. But can forgiveness be taught? Can she stop blaming herself for not knowing, in spite of her efforts, what was on the mind of her dead soldier?

## PROFESSIONAL REFLECTIONS

During the wars in Iraq and Afghanistan, the soldier suicide rate increased to a level surpassing the civilian suicide rate. At one point, more soldiers were killing themselves than were being killed by the enemy. The Army as a whole, just like this soldier, did not see it coming either. The Army, too, began looking.

They found the usual factors. Suicides are associated with mental health problems, impulsivity, and drug or alcohol use and combat stress. "Dear John letters" from a girlfriend are a factor. But they also found that not all soldiers who committed suicide had been in combat.

The suicide rate is so high in some smaller units that individual soldiers "fear" it is infectious. Studies confirm empirically what soldiers report anecdotally. Nearly one half of our veterans knew someone who killed him or herself, and 65 percent of that group knew more than one victim (Ursano, 2017).

That fact alone makes a soldier more likely to think about and/or commit suicide. The Army studied the work environment and the communication surrounding suicides in these high-rate units. The Army suspects that how leaders and the soldiers' peers deal with suicide attempts and deaths is a factor in this contagion.

I believe underlying these numbers is unresolved grief. Soldiers bond in cohesive units in which they pledge to protect one another with their own lives. There is an emotional blurring of self and other. Combat is a communal experience, but grief work often is not. When the other dies, it feels emotionally as if "it should have been me. When the other needed me, I was not there." Guilt generates more grief. Grief suffered alone can be so painful, make one so angry, that killing another seems the only way to relieve the pain. Killing oneself can become the ultimate loyal act.

Telling this soldier all that information would not help. She knows it and did everything she could have done. Her feelings of responsibility probably stemmed from the early losses in her life for which she inexplicably blamed herself. She needs to forgive herself for something for which she is not morally responsible. Forgiveness, like grief, must be a collective experience.

# PART II

# WEAPONS

CHAPTER FIVE

# IEDS—IMPROVISED EXPLOSIVE DEVICES

### *"Who Knew Changing Diapers Could Be Such A Problem?"*

Trauma affects different parts of the brain and therefore the mind. The hippocampus is a databank for memory. It organizes memories according to time and place and connects them to emotions. The amygdala monitors the memory and emotional input and instructs the body to respond. In PTSD, the hippocampus gets the time and place confused and stores the memory as a fragment not as a whole. The amygdala may perceive the way the memory and emotional data are mixed as dangerous. Individuals with PTSD have no "off switch," so a perceived threat leads to dysregulation between the hippocampus and the amygdala. These parts of the brain are overwhelmed, and so they signal distress to the body and the mind to "know" there is danger.

While working at Walter Reed, I have learned that servicemen and women experience trauma in many different ways. There seems to be no end to the complexity. Everyone has a different limit as to how much trauma he or she can tolerate, but when experienced it is always unique. Two recent examples brought this "uniqueness" to my attention. One I read about and the other I listened to.

I read a former colleague's report (Lacoursiere, 2017) of a patient who was involved in a nighttime landing of tanks on shore. As an infantryman, he was guiding the offloading of the tanks from special landing craft. Somehow, under reduced light and adverse conditions, the situation deteriorated.

Suddenly, one of the rackety monstrosities was right in front of him. He fell to the ground and lay as flat, straight, and motionless as he could, parallel to the approaching machine's treads. He was terrified between the tracks as the tank clanged over him, thankfully without causing physical injury.

He survived physically unscathed. Many years later, the soldier had back problems unrelated to this experience. Referred for an MRI, he became "paralyzed" with fear. The potential claustrophobia and "notorious clamor" of the MRI overwhelmed his brain, his body, and his mind.

In the other incident, I listened to a forty-year-old soldier for a number of months. He'd had attention deficit disorder since elementary school yet functioned well. He spent about twenty years in the Army as a military police officer and had a few deployments. The medication he takes allows him to be appropriately attentive at his job and concentrate well. He has an older son, and his wife was expecting. He is now considering retirement and possibly moving to the area where his wife was born.

Recently, he went there for an interview for a civilian job on a local police force. Full disclosure: His father-in-law is the chief of police and the service member has twenty years of experience in the military police. The tests went well, the security clearance will take some time, but he is optimistic he will be offered a position. The transition from military to civilian life is complicated, but he is taking many appropriate advance-planning steps. He and his wife seem to be in agreement, and their life is going well.

About two months following the birth of his daughter, he returned for an appointment. Distressed, disheveled and distraught, he said he could not sleep. I made some inane comment about how the sleeping habits of young babies can be hard on "older" parents.

"No," he said, "not that. It is the nightmares, of gathering up body parts." Having no record of these symptoms, I asked him to explain. He told me that it had happened a little when his son was born, but that the birth of his daughter had triggered nightly multiple nightmares of his deployments. I asked him to explain.

His military police job in Iraq had been to secure the streets and ensure safe passage for both civilians and the military. IEDs used by insurgents to kill almost two-thirds of our soldiers were a constant problem. IEDs may have conventional military explosives, but they are used in unconventional ways such as roadside bombs attached to an "unseen" detonating mechanism.

One day, he watched two Iraqi families packed into a small Toyota Corolla drive by on their way to the grocery store or for religious worship. As they passed under a nearby bridge, their vehicle suddenly exploded. Vehicle and body parts flew everywhere. His job of ensuring security now became one of collecting body parts into body bags. Collecting fragments of children was especially difficult.

And now, while changing diapers on his newborn, handling those small, flexible, vulnerable body parts, this service member is reminded of that awful work his job required. He ponders, "One moment a happy family, the next moment just body parts." There is no explanation. "Their car just drove over the wrong spot."

Those of us fortunate enough to have children change diapers—not always pleasant, but it is part of being a parent. This soldier who served on our behalf has a much more difficult job being a parent.

Changing diapers or getting an MRI should not be so difficult.

## PROFESSIONAL REFLECTION

The US military, designed originally to deliver overwhelming force, has found itself instead fighting insurgencies in Iraq and Afghanistan. IEDs are conventionally made bombs used in unconventional warfare by terrorist organizations to counteract the asymmetry in forces. In previous wars, booby traps and landmines were used. In Iraq and Afghanistan, as opposed to Vietnam, almost twice as many soldiers, up to 66 percent of all casualties, are killed by IEDs.

This soldier retired with no physical injury. Yet, witnessing the explosion of the IED and the destruction of a civilian family, combined with the collection of body parts, leaves him with intrusive memories reminding him of his service to our country. Some soldiers continue suffering even while carrying out the most mundane daily tasks of living.

# CHAPTER SIX

# SUICIDAL BOMBER: UP FRONT AND PERSONAL

The first scheduled patient was quite late. When he arrived, his appointment time was half gone. The nurse at the remote location said he was having difficulty completing the information packet. Ordinarily in a situation like this, the bureaucracy just closes down the appointment and the service member is rescheduled for another week.

I was ambivalent. I always try to make accommodations, but if I were to see him it would throw off the schedule for the entire day. It is not just me, but everyone after him would be inconvenienced. Upon reflection, I realized these visits are always important if not urgent and told the nurse to bring in the new patient.

"Why are you here and how can I help?" is the usual first question. This young man had just been transferred to a new base and was seeking a psychiatrist because his prior psychotherapy had been so helpful. An interesting chief complaint! After multiple trials, he had found an antidepressant that worked and additional medication for his memory problems. Among his more pressing long-term problems were significant short-term memory difficulties and associated reading problems. How had these problems come about?

He explained that he had been in a convoy while deployed. He was several vehicles from the lead and riding in one of the passenger seats. He watched as the trucks in front of him passed the cars parked on the side of the road. Suddenly, a parked car moved directly in front of his vehicle. The explosion wounded the members of his vehicle, and he lost consciousness for a brief period.

When he awoke, it was clear that he was the most able-bodied survivor to drive his "buddies" for medical attention. In spite of his wounds, he was able to position himself in the driver's seat. Attempting to restart the engine, he realized he could not see through the windshield. The suicide bomber had been "liquefied" and the remains were like a paste that covered the front of his vehicle, obscuring any vision. He literally had to scrape the remains off the windshield before they could proceed. Luckily everyone survived (except the bomber).

My patient has PTSD and traumatic brain injury, the source of his short-term memory and reading problems. Several years have passed and he seems remarkably "upbeat." He has received appropriate treatment. "A friend" helped him relearn how to read and take notes simultaneously, which helps his comprehension. He has learned how to be more disciplined, orderly, and focused than previously.

The Army suggested he be medically retired. His physical and behavioral health injuries certainly qualify him for that. He refused. He maintains that he can perform his job albeit a bit more slowly than before. Put to the test, he passed.

"Why do you want to stay?" I asked. He responded, "I have a lot to offer the Army and those who come after me. I have experience, wisdom, and good judgment to pass on to those who follow."

We all hit roadblocks in life, an impasse here or there. A failed marriage, the death of a family member, a child with a severe impairment, but a suicide bomber? Ironically, this service member has experienced all four of the above.

He and his former wife have two children. He describes his ex-spouse as a wonderful mother just a "lousy wife." His younger sister died in childbirth. As a result, his mother worries "excessively" over him. His younger child has significant mental retardation. He describes her as "high functioning" in school. He has a positive perspective on each of these experiences.

Did these prior tragedies somehow prepare him for being hit by a suicide bomber? Is he able to adjust more easily because he has had to accommodate to significant tragedy? He lost a sister, a wife, and has an impaired child. He stills gets nauseous when exposed to certain smells. He still focuses on what he can give to others. He is amused by his mother's worry about him. He appears to be doing just fine.

I will wait to see a guy like this anytime.

Between the first and second visits, I kept thinking about him. His adjustment seemed too good to be true. He returned stating that he had problems falling asleep—that moment when by yourself, in bed trying to relax, one lets go. He first became fearful of falling asleep after the suicide bomber experience.

I decided to jump into that abyss with him; after all, that's my job. "What do you think about as you are trying to fall asleep?" I asked. "What if there is no God?" he responded. With such a leap in context, it just seemed natural to ask him what he thought about his suicide bomber. He became speechless and silent. Maybe I had gone too far.

Finally, he was able to say that he had never been asked that question. So many thoughts were racing through his mind that he was speechless. First, he wanted to attack the bomber. Then came the questions. How could the bomber disguise himself as a civilian and hide in the shopping center with all the innocent people? There is a higher moral code to how a war is fought, he protested. There is no honor in fighting the way the bomber fought. This soldier had been the commander of his unit, and after the bombing he felt the need "to appear strong for his men." He never told any of them about his reaction. Was there any discussion of the moral methods of war?

His sleep problems can be treated medically. The great yet simple insight developed extensively since World War II is that talking about these traumatic matters in a systematic way is helpful.

What about the moral injuries? How we fight and how they fight and if we should be fighting? This young man is speechless at the question. And for the most part, so is the United States.

## PROFESSIONAL REFLECTIONS

This soldier's story presents several issues: asymmetrical warfare in the form of IEDs and suicide bombers, how one processes loss and killing, how one fights wars honorably, and whether one should continue fighting.

Dr. Madelyn Hsiao-Rei Hicks' report (2011), written for the Rand Corporation, stated that suicide bombings have increased since the advent of modern international terrorism began in 1968. In the ten years after the beginning of the war in Iraq, suicide bombers killed 12,284 Iraqi civilians and wounded 30,644.

A response to asymmetrical warfare, suicide bombing is inexpensive, effective, and designed to rip the fabric of trust and predictability out of society. Israel and the United States have technologically superior warfare. Bruce Hoffman in *The Atlantic* (2003) states that Al-Qaeda and others allege that both countries have citizens who are materialistic, lazy, and are no longer willing to sacrifice lives to defend their national interests. Furthermore, the report stated that Israel was considered a testing ground for terrorism before suicide bombing becomes more prevalent in the US. Israel is responding to terrorism and does have required national service for all citizens in the Israel Defense Forces.

International terrorists are counting on the 99 percent of Americans not being like this soldier. Experts predict it is only a matter of time before more suicide bombers operate within the United States. Americans could learn a great deal about coping with and surviving tragedy as well as being citizen volunteers by talking with soldiers like this one. Preparation for terrorism may become important to ensure the future integrity of our society already fractured by the current tribalism. We may find ourselves relying on the example of soldiers like this one for guidance.

This soldier, a victim of a suicide bomber, has a traumatic brain injury (TBI) manifested by short-term memory problems, poor attention and organizational skills, and difficulty reading. He continues to serve because of his motivation and his self-proclaimed wisdom, experience, and judgment.

He fulfills Aristotle's definition of a tragic narrative, a miserable suffering person who has experienced a death of a family member, among other things. And out of his Greek-like tragedy, he searches for God and a stronger bond with his fellow men. He resolves to fight war honorably.

First, in his rage, he wanted to attack the bomber. Then he experienced bewilderment at how the bomber could do this to innocent people! There was no discussion with his men of their shared grief and loss. He proceeds stoically and honorably.

He poses the central question in asymmetrical warfare. Our side has overwhelming conventional firepower, so why does the enemy not want to fight in our manner? If they fight in our advantageous manner, they will lose. So, they leverage their disadvantage by fighting in what we define as a dishonorable manner.

Our military has been slow in providing official guidance to this soldier and his unit on how to fight a counterinsurgency. "The updated field manual for counterinsurgency, . . . the playbook for operations . . . was issued only in December 2006, some five years after the first troops deployed to Afghanistan" (Sherman, 2011, 76).

These conditions—IEDs, suicidal bombers, multiple deployments, unclear guidelines of engagement—put stress on group cohesion and thinking. The principle of altruism, shared protection, and honorable behavior can, under stress, be eroded. Loss of members to unfair fighting can be perceived as signs of dishonor to a unit and disloyalty to principles of war.

Mutual loyalty and protection of the group from loss can now, under stress, lead to revenge for the loss of a member. The principled behavior of honorable service members can regress. Soldiers who defer grief in battle, whether from manly virtue or no leisure time for grieving, may fight more vengefully. Anger is a useful tool to activate the mind for combat. Unchecked anger, taking pleasure in killing, does not win the "hearts and minds" of the people. Anger unhampered by grief risks not just loss of life but loss of one's humanity. Close monitoring of one's emotions are facilitated by rules of engagement.

The counterinsurgency manual states that the enemy is often unseen, not wearing uniforms and mingles with civilians. Understanding the local customs and politics may be as important as, or more important, than maintaining superior firepower. Under these conditions, overwhelming force, fueled by unchecked anger, may be counterproductive. Killing legitimate enemies as well as innocent civilians may paradoxically make a combat unit less safe.

We citizens expect our soldiers in war to play by the honorable rules despite enemy behavior. We citizens, possibly expecting less of ourselves, are rapidly beginning not to play by the rules while engaging in civilian strife. Patriotism requires vigorous debate while playing by the rules.

This soldier, a victim of suicide bombing, resolves to continue to act honorably. We citizens, modeling ourselves on his behavior, should not do less in our civic discussion/life.

# CHAPTER SEVEN

# *THE HURT LOCKER* AND MAN'S BEST FRIEND

The movie *The Hurt Locker*, about a bomb disposal team, illustrated one way the military deals with how the nature of war has changed. The Explosive Ordnance Disposal Team in the movie clears the field of IEDs and landmines that are now more prevalent in combat and noncombat areas. In my telepsychiatry work, I met one of these men whose job it was to detect IEDs.

This soldier volunteered to be an explosive detection dog handler not because he was unusually brave but because he had been left behind. Injured during training just before his deployment, his unit deployed without him. When he recovered, he was unable to get orders to rejoin his unit. He voluntarily trained as an explosive detection dog handler with the understanding that he would be able to rejoin his unit in the field. It never happened.

After completion of his ordnance detection training, he was deployed. Attached to one brigade, the soldier was loaned out to others for routine clearance of culverts, choke points, and cache and mountain searches. Still, he never found his unit.

In retrospect, the soldier had signs of the invisible traumatic brain injury (TBI), a condition indicated, among other things, by memory problems, headaches, and difficulty thinking. Before the last deployment as an explosive detection dog handler, the soldier had prior deployments in the regular infantry. Indeed, he had been exposed previously to IEDs and suffered brain damage no one else had detected. This invisible injury may have contributed to his lack of knowledge of the risks his duties as an explosive detection dog handler might involve. Nor did he imagine the increased risk his military occupational specialty (MOS) had for violent injury and death. "I didn't do my research into dog team casualties," he explained.

Apparently, he did not know that nearly 45,000 Americans have been evacuated from both the Iraqi and Afghanistan wars for injury from combat wounds. Nor had he heard that those casualties include over 1,350 amputees and another 6,800 with limbs so damaged they imperil the soldiers' functioning. He later realized that the percentage of dog team handlers who come back having lost limbs or in body bags is significantly higher than those sustaining injury in a regular infantry brigade.

I asked him what the experience was like.

"Pretty nerve-racking," he replied. "But my work was important stuff! I found things that could have been walked on. And I saved some lives." He further explained, "There was really no one to talk to about this stuff except my dog, and he was my closest friend."

"What happened to your dog?" I asked.

"He was 'recycled' to another soldier."

Remarkably, this soldier showed no signs of physical injury. No lost limbs. Although at greater risk for physical harm, he completed his tour without visible injury. Yet, he never found *his unit*. It was this strong desire to reunite with his unit that caused him to volunteer for this dangerous job as an explosive detection dog handler. His unit was like an emotional magnet for him, and yet it engaged him in a big risk that, in the end, provided him with no reunion.

It is a fact that the way wars are fought today has changed. It obviously remains lethal and violent, but the strategy for inflicting injury, death, and disability is different. Bombs, and especially suicide bombers, do more damage than bullets now. The damage—paradoxically—is both more visible and more invisible.

Our enemy now relies less on bullets, too, and more on IEDs. Not only does this change require modification in our fighting strategy, it causes a change in the nature of injury and disability in our soldiers. Suicide bombers, essentially mobile IEDs as well as stationary IEDs, traumatize and kill our soldiers. More service members survive injuries than in prior wars but with greater physical trauma (multiple amputations). And more survive with the invisible trauma, traumatic brain injury. Many recent *New York Times* and CBS *60 Minutes* news pieces suggest that length and number of deployments and incidence of TBI may contribute to the increased incidence of suicides in current veterans as compared to suicides among Vietnam veterans. Are these present-day IEDs helping to kill our soldiers slowly over time?

I talked with the soldier in our telepsychiatry session about missing his regular infantry unit, and I also asked if he missed his dog.

"I have no desire to pet dogs. They have lost their luster," he said. This man lost his friends and his dog. His service saved lives and because of his TBI, he may have lost much of his own life. His service kept other service members safer.

We know many of these soldiers go to war, return home, and look healthy. In the past, if soldiers looked physically fit, they could continue their work. As a society, we need to be more mindful and knowledgeable about the effects of battle on soldiers' minds.

This soldier firmly believes his work protected other soldiers. Has this soldier's service affected us in any way? Do we want to know what soldiers go through to perform their service? If these soldiers act as our proxies, what more do we expect from them? Maybe we should expect more of ourselves?

## PROFESSIONAL REFLECTIONS

America has demonstrated that it can win wars of overwhelming force. Hence, the mindset of our enemies has changed. Their attitudinal shift is reflected in their war technology. The increased use of IEDs and suicidal bombers (mobile IEDs) changed the nature of fighting and of injuries suffered by our troops. More soldiers survive combat but suffer greater physical and psychological damage.

IEDs are deployed in various ways and locations, designed to fragment armored vehicles and human bodies as well as the functioning of the human brain. Their capacity to fragment the functioning of the brain allows their effect to persist over time. Autopsies of soldiers with IED-induced traumatic brain injury indicate that brain tissue has been microfractured, separating brain tissue from its blood supply. It is not a broken bone but a broken brain. Over time, soldiers, who have pledged not to kill themselves, find themselves tormented with pain and dysfunction and do commit suicide. Soldiers and families have understood that they may be physically injured during wartime. Less well anticipated is the fact that an IED injury might continue to kill a brain slowly over time.

The surprise attack nature of these type of weapons has increased from a low of 3-4 percent deaths in WWII and Korea, 11 percent deaths and 17 percent injuries in Vietnam, increasing to 67 percent of casualties in Iraq and Afghanistan (*Achilles in Vietnam*, 32–34).

This enemy deception and unpredictability has changed our mindset and unfortunately our minds. A soldier may survive physically, but TBI continues, as the brain can slowly deteriorate. Furthermore, the unpredictability of an attack can lead to a distrust of social order.

Soldier/author Thomas Brennan, who suffered a TBI, says in his book, *Shooting Ghosts*, "People love to tell me I look fine. My wounds are invisible to most people but visible to me." He further describes the moral wounds of war, wounds that arise from what soldiers do to themselves and their enemies, all fellow human beings. Brennan asserts that one never gets over trauma but finds a way to get through it. His wounded soul is mended in part by the collective redemptive experience of co-authorship of his book with photojournalist Finbarr O'Reilly.

Anger and rage reactions can overwhelm underlying grief about the experience, trapping individuals in the isolation of trauma. Their joint narration of the book is one example of the importance of communalizing the war experience. Survivors must not be left alone to metabolize grief and trauma within themselves. Americans—family, friends, neighbors, and even strangers—must connect to soldiers in informal and formal ways to hear their stories.

This soldier, an explosive detection dog handler, lost his combat friends and his dog. Yet, his service saved lives and because of his TBI, he may have lost much of his own life. His service kept other service members safer. When you see him on the street, he deserves your connection beyond, "Thank you for your service."

# PART III

# DEALING WITH DEATH

# CHAPTER EIGHT

# "GIVING UP ON COMPASSION WORKS?"

This service member's pain preceded her entrance into the room. From outside, I could hear it in her voice when she said, "I am not going to do it." The secretary called ahead and said the service member refused to complete the required paperwork and asked if that would disqualify her for the visit. It usually does. I decided to proceed anyway.

A young woman with a disarming smile appeared. Her presentation did not fit with the phone call description. "My provider got reassigned. I am just here to get my medication renewal," she said. As I reviewed her list of medicines, I surmised she had some serious problems, probably PTSD.

We began talking about her history and none of the "preliminary hostility" was evident. She was pleasant and cooperative. Yet, she recounted a more than ten-year history of serious depression, anxiety, nightmares, social withdrawal, and isolation. This history is frequently recited by someone injured during deployment.

She denied ever having been physically injured during a deployment. I asked, nevertheless, more about the deployments.

She listed several extended deployments to all the battle zones and wars established by the the United States during the past fifteen years. "No physical injury," she repeated.

"But you must have seen a lot of trauma?" I hesitantly asked.

"I sent a lot of soldiers home with a flag," she responded.

For a while, I continued talking, but my mind was trying to figure out why she gave them flags. Even after eight years in this work, I can be a little slow to see death.

This soldier simply wanted her medication renewed. Nevertheless, I asked her what type of job provided her the opportunity to drape a flag over each dead soldier's coffin. "Witnessing trauma," she replied. "I assembled the body parts." She talked about how she was prepared for seeing death. She read books and studied about it. She went to operating rooms to witness trauma and trauma surgery. She prepared in every way she could imagine. "I forced myself to be *part* of the trauma," she said. I asked her if it helped. "Not at all," was her response.

"Intellectually, one can prepare, but emotionally it is another story," she added. She went on, noting that she had tried preparing to see trauma and death, but she was not prepared for the reaction of medical personnel to the process of dying. I asked her what she meant.

"Watching two and one-half hours of terminal labored breathing gets to people," she said. She saw some irritated and overworked medics yell, "Stop breathing" at one dying patient so they could get on to the next dying person.

In retrospect, she tried to evaluate each case to see what could have been done better. During the process, she worked at trying to make herself numb. Her eventual solution was to give up on being compassionate. "If I had no compassion, dealing with death became easier." As I listened, her expression suggested that her mind had just left the room. I asked if she were back on the battlefield. "I can be right there in that moment, right now, right now," said this soldier who gave up on compassion. One of the cardinal signs of PTSD is re-experiencing the past while living in the present. I could see her going back and forth while she tried to talk about it.

Knowing the importance of talking about these experiences, I asked with whom she speaks. "I can talk with civilian friends," she said, "but they do not understand. I can talk with my husband, but he does not want to hear it."

"What did you see?" I asked. She described bodies and parts destroyed beyond recognition. Her job was to identify them and bag them together, but there was no way to know who they were. She described her promotion into this job because she had showed that she could do it without compassion. All the male soldiers cried too much.

Before this initial interview was over, I had to ask if she had ever attempted suicide. "Too many times to count," she responded. "It is always on my mind. But just the sissy stuff like overdosing with pills and cutting wrists. Nothing serious."

Before she left, she said that she had been referred for a Medical Evaluation Board in which the military service determines if one has a particular diagnosis and if it is service connected. If so, one is entitled to a medical retirement with benefits. This soldier had recounted to me some of the worst trauma I have heard. She demonstrated involuntarily her PTSD symptoms right in front of me. She said the board had agreed that she had PTSD but that the cause was childhood trauma. *No service connected medical retirement.* I said, "That is ridiculous." "That is what my other provider said also," she responded.

I guess the United States Army also gave up on compassion.

I asked her to come back and she agreed.

## PROFESSIONAL REFLECTIONS

Immediately, one thinks, *Can't a letter be written to rectify this error in judgment?* Apparently not! The Army has decided. She can, however, revisit the service-connected medical issue with the Veterans Administration. There will be another opportunity to give appropriate meaning to her service.

But what about the meaning she gave to the careful management of all those bodies? Subsequent visits revealed just how compassionately this soldier did care for the bodies and by that compassionate concern did give some measure of meaning to their deaths. Despite her intense personal symptoms, she was enormously proud of her contribution to the memory and service of her fallen comrades. She spoke of maintaining this pride in her heart despite the bureaucratic failure to recognize her service-connected symptoms.

I could not help but think that this soldier had given the last full measure of devotion to her fallen comrades while our bureaucracy failed to do the same for her.

Archibald MacLeish, while serving as Librarian of Congress, wrote the following poem for a memorial service.

"The Young Dead Soldiers"

They say, "We leave you our deaths. Give them their meaning.
We were young, they say. We have died; remember us."

The young dead soldiers do not speak.
Nevertheless, they are heard in the still houses:
who has not heard them?

They have a silence that speaks for them at night
and when the clock counts.

They say: We were young. We have died.
Remember us.

They say: We have done what we could
but until it is finished it is not done.

They say: We have given our lives but until it is finished
no one can know what our lives gave.

They say: Our deaths are not ours: they are yours,
they will mean what you make them.

They say: Whether our lives and our deaths were for
peace and a new hope or for nothing we cannot say,
it is you who must say this.

We leave you our deaths. Give them their meaning.
We were young, they say. We have died; remember us.

**The poem asks us to think about the sacrifices made by soldiers on our behalf and what meaning we will give to their service and death.**

# CHAPTER NINE
# FORGIVENESS

Physicians generally like the people they treat. I have enjoyed most of the people with whom I have worked but not all. If you really do not like someone, it often becomes difficult to be helpful.

I have seen one soldier many times whom I did not like. While she was likable, I did not like the experience of working with her. It took me too long to figure out that she was not the problem so much as how I felt while treating her. So, I was not able to help her very much and that made me feel helpless. Only much later did I piece together each of our parts in the medical relationship.

She had served more than one tour under difficult circumstances. Her career was long and productive. Afterward, she had nightmares, depression, anxiety, panic attacks, and fainting spells. Mostly, however, she suffered from an overwhelming sense of helplessness under pressure. She just did not *seem* to be able to do anything about her situation. Nothing I did or offered improved her condition substantially. Most troubling was the fainting spells she experienced. She would pass out, losing consciousness under unpredictable circumstances. She had the appropriate medical and neurological workups and no cause could be found. She could no longer safely work or drive a car because she would pass out without warning.

Physicians always think there has to be a medical explanation. With panic attacks, physicians invariably think that the patient must be thinking about uncomfortable things that prompt the anxiety, which then generalizes and becomes out of control. More recently, a whole body of knowledge has shown that individuals have a biochemical storm that may account for their panic, and it may not be related to what they were thinking. Medications administered before or after the experience can alter the experience and calm them down. The experience does not have to stem from psychological causes. It may be stimulated by a real life event that the mind pairs with some past troubling experience. An event so simple—as driving down the interstate under a bridge—can trigger a panic attack that reminds the mind automatically of a patrol while deployed in Iraq or Afghanistan.

I tried to help this solider examine her life and figure out what was happening in her mind before she passed out. In short, we never got anywhere, and I did not like working with her because the sessions went nowhere.

One day, she came in and was excited. She seemed relieved. She said she was beginning to think she knew what the cause was. She had never told anyone her story. Working as a medic on a medical evacuation helicopter can be stressful. On this day in question, she had worked on multiple evacuations from sun up to sun down under dangerous conditions. After the last evacuation, her exhausted crew lifted off for their home base. As they were returning home, she saw a human figure pointing something at the helicopter, and it flashed several times. Assuming they were taking "hostile fire," she urged evasive action.

The next morning, rested and reflecting, she suddenly realized the flash was from a device given to soldiers seeking help. The device was designed to emit a light only upward and not horizontally so that the surrounding enemy could not see it. The soldier she directed her helicopter crew to leave was not an enemy directing hostile fire.

Rather, that soldier was a comrade seeking their help. The thought of having abandoned this soldier left her feeling completely helpless.

This story was a like a big NEON SIGN in front of me flashing "helplessness."

Maybe this was not so much a medical problem as a moral problem. She did the wrong thing—not through any fault of her own—but she made the wrong judgment or decision. Only in retrospect did her intellectual mind know that! The emotional mind does not work that way. Armed with new information, it tends to hold us responsible—not for the facts as presented at the time but for the facts as you know them now. That is a battle that cannot be won. Only forgiveness works.

A poetic rendition of Psalm 51 may be an appropriate reflection: "Speak to me in words that release me." Medically, I did not know how to do that for this soldier. Fortunately, she went to a hospital specializing in PTSD. The hospitalization was helpful in terms of treatment, but more help may have come from the experience of meeting some infantrymen in group therapy. She only saw failure that "ate me alive." They, however, saw a heroine who, on a particular day, had saved many lives. "We were deployed at different times, but what we saw and felt was the same and so it became a shared experience," she reported.

Finding a way to forgive oneself is the key, or finding someone *else* who will forgive you can be just as much of a key. This conundrum is more moral than medical. Veteran Thomas Gibbons-Neff (2015) reflected this idea when he wrote in *The Washington Post*:

*"Recognizing moral injury isn't so much about how the country understands its veterans; rather it is about how veterans understand themselves... and it's also about reconnecting with a moral community feeling connected to your fellow man."*

Since hearing her story, it is interesting how much my attitude toward this soldier has changed, how much I look forward to seeing her. She is feeling better, fainting less frequently. Maybe the change in me is due to what I now see that we have in common: the ability to forgive ourselves of our own mistakes, for that is part of what it means to be human.

## PROFESSIONAL REFLECTIONS

Service members fight for cause and for comrades. Medics serve maybe even more so for comrades than cause. This soldier spent a long day rescuing comrades. One last final call for help she misinterpreted, only realizing the mistake upon reflection on another day.

She was paralyzed by guilt over a decisive act, a failure to save a comrade. It was a decision she could not repair. The ambiguity of the effects of her action—did the abandoned solider die or not?—made her situation all the more complicated. This situation is like facing death, not one's own but in someone else. All of us have struggled with the question, "If only I could have or should have . . ." Failure is part of what makes us human. Collective understanding of our condition can foster forgiveness.

She presented her helplessness to me cloaked with many other symptoms. I was unable to recognize the source of her helplessness, just as she had failed to recognize the source of the flashing light. We were helpless together until she began one day to tell her story.

Then, like a neon sign, it became obvious. The helplessness she was acting out in our sessions and was unable to talk about or describe reflected the helplessness she experienced in not saving the last soldier. Her paralysis hindered my ability to be helpful to her. I felt helpless and did not like the experience of being with her. My contribution to our shared problem, paradoxically, was in part me trying to be helpful. I was focused on what triggered her anxiety symptoms, reducing the nightmares, and reducing her depression. By being so focused on "short term" issues, I failed to see the overarching one: She suffered from an overwhelming sense of helplessness under pressure. "Sophocles teaches . . . the uncompensated physical agony humans can undergo as the result of mistake" (Sherman, 2011,100).

Finding her narrative was critical. Her solution was more moral than medical. She had to find an appropriate way to grieve this unintentional error. She spent hours in a group with infantrymen deployed at a different time and in a different place. Yet, the similarity of their experiences led to a bonding through mutual grief. These were comrades who once again were saving one another's lives. This group became her moral community.

Grieving is an essential part of war. "What is at risk in war is not just a loss of life but goodness" (Sherman, 2011, 84).

America must create not only more spaces for service but also for acknowledgment of appropriate grief regarding war. We as a people at war need to include soldiers and ourselves in a larger moral community, one that has suffered but is trying to find goodness in all of us as we dedicate ourselves to the common good. There are multiple opportunities in book clubs, libraries, school rooms, town meetings, Memorial Day services, churches, synagogues, and YMCAs for citizens to listen, learn, and foster healing.

## CHAPTER TEN

# I DID NOT KILL ANY HUMANS, JUST GOOKS

During my private practice seeing civilian patients, I frequently worked with couples and families. As often as possible, I tried to interview both members of a marital pair. There is always value in obtaining another view of a clinical problem. I followed the same procedure while working with service members. Sometimes, both spouses were service members. On rare occasions, both spouses had been deployed to the same location at different times. Such was the case with the Smiths. Sarah Smith went first, and John Smith went second.

Within her leadership position, Dr. Sarah Smith was exposed to a lot of trauma. As a trauma surgeon, she worked in the emergency room and intensive care unit. Most of her contact with patients was short term. Injuries were triaged. What injuries she could repair, she did. What injuries she could not resolve were evacuated. She had no long-term contact with injured individuals. She returned to the United States, retired, and continued caring for her family.

Her husband, John Smith, deployed a month after her return and was sent to the location where she had been a military surgeon. Sarah told her husband not to worry about this deployment. There was a great deal of combat nearby, but he would be safe. Despite the frequent shelling and bombings, John remained physically safe. Shortly after arrival, he learned a college classmate had committed suicide. Somewhat later, one of his deployed colleagues killed herself. Midway through his deployment, a field grade officer on the verge of promotion took his own life. John was unnerved by these events. He began thinking a great deal about the value of a life.

Dr. John Smith had intimate contact with his patients, many of whom were our soldiers and many of whom were enemy soldiers. He ran a rehabilitation center, focusing on occupational and physical therapy. Some of the enemy were "high value" prisoners. He was obligated to take good care of them in part because of the information they might provide. His care involved daily physical and emotional contact. He developed personal relationships and was concerned about their welfare. When rehabilitated and debriefed, these enemy combatants were sometimes released. He knew that the rehabbed prisoners might be assassinated by their colleagues as soon as they left the compound. Some were. These enemy soldiers often begged not to be let go. They knew, as did Dr. Smith, that the enemy would consider the patient debriefing as a betrayal. Dr. Smith had no control over their release.

He also knew that some of the captured enemy were quite dangerous. He ministered to them under perilous conditions in which he had to monitor his own safety. Alone in an unguarded moment, he could be injured himself. Needing to help someone who might in turn injure you can lead to a very ambivalent relationship.

Upon his return home, his wife found him to be a different person—emotionally distant, hypervigilant, avoiding crowds, experiencing nightmares, and frequently anxious. He was sleepy in the daytime and wished that somehow he would die. Pressed by his wife to discuss his deployment, he became tearful. She knew what the deployment had been like. She had been there, but it was not what her husband was describing. Sarah had not been there in the same way John had, and she could not understand his reaction. Marital conflict ensued, compounding his condition.

Two soldiers, one marriage, deployed in the same place experienced totally different reactions. Medically, it might be easy to explain away these differences as genetics, life history, different physiology, or different time frames. I told them, however, that I thought a major factor in their conflict was the different relationship they each had with the enemy.

A soldier appearing in the PBS Burns and Novick series, *The Vietnam War,* summed it up best by saying, "I did not kill any humans, only gooks." In other words, he had no relationship with the enemy. After one dehumanizes the enemy, the rest of the war is easier.

John Smith was unable to dehumanize the enemy. He literally *cared* for the enemy and was concerned about his or her welfare. Emotionally metabolizing the experience was fraught with conflicting feelings. This problem was not shared by his wife, who had no such long-term personal relationship with the enemy.

His reaction was similar to a North Vietnamese soldier quoted in the PBS series. The enemy soldier said the Americans seem like us: courageous, loyal, and really concerned about one another. Americans do not abandon their fallen soldiers. They go back for them—a behavior that we also show.

Caring about the enemy is not new to the wars in Vietnam, Iraq, and Afghanistan. The behavior is part of a long tradition. Perhaps the most famous example of mutual caring for the enemy was the World War I Christmas truce. Along the Western front on Christmas Day, 1914, over 100,000 British, Belgian, and French troops mixed with German soldiers. It began in the trenches first with the Germans singing Christmas carols, then the British or Belgians sang from the other side, and then finally they came up over the wires to join in singing "O Come, All Ye Faithful" in English and Latin. Graham Williams of the Fifth London Rifle Brigade said, "Well, this is really a most extraordinary thing—two nations both singing the same carol in the middle of a war."

During the American Civil War, over 700,000 individuals died. President Lincoln spoke as the war was coming to an end, "With malice toward none, with charity for all, with firmness in the right as God gives us to see the right." One nation, a house divided, at war which tried to find a way to live with one another.

Dr. Smith has found it helpful to know that his care and concern for the enemy, the behavior complicating his current life, is part of a long and honorable tradition. He is not alone. Not everyone finds it easy to dehumanize our fellow enemies. As John understands himself better, so does his wife. Perhaps even we, our nation, may understand better some of war's complexities as well.

## PROFESSIONAL REFLECTIONS

So, what are some of those personal and societal complexities of war? Soldiers often say, "I was just doing my job." These two soldiers, husband and wife, had very different responses to doing their jobs. Their different reactions raise the question as to what exactly is the job of war. Who defines and creates the individual jobs and the overall goal of war, and what difference does that make?

Our leaders, our elected representatives, on our behalf often shape our views of war. They define the enemy and determine if we will have a large-scale military operation or a smaller-scale counterinsurgency effort or even nuclear war. Essentially, the president designs a national political strategy that he or she believes is unachievable without war. Based on the overall goal developed by the president and his staff, the military planners fill in the military details to achieve the national goal. All this planning is done on our behalf as we the people of the United States go to war with our enemy, another group of people.

Wars generally arise out of a political failure to resolve a difference between two groups of people or two countries. These differences frequently are about territory or political systems. Usually, it involves taking over some of the enemy's territory or defending one's own territory. Or it may be about overthrowing the enemy's political system. Basically, we go to war because our leaders and their leaders cannot politically and diplomatically work out the perceived differences (McPherson, 70-75).

Individual soldiers function better when their military job fits appropriately into the national strategy. Killing the enemy is necessary to recover territory or to defend one's own territory. Soldiers function much better when the goals are clear. Overthrowing a political system requires not only killing the enemy but winning the hearts and minds of the people—presenting a delicate balance with less clarity.

If we think of our enemy as less than us, it is easier to go to war. If we think of them as "gooks," "krauts," "wops," "guineas," "axis of evil," "rocket man," or "godless communists," and so on, it is easier to kill them. But when they know we disrespect them, it is harder to win their hearts and minds.

Dr. John Smith's job was complex. He was bewildered by the fact that he did not always see prisoners as the enemy. Some of his patients were also dangerous people. The job our soldiers face in winning the hearts and minds of the people is complicated. Those Afghan soldiers that our soldiers train may be friendly during training, but they may become part of enemy attacks after our training.

A substantial number of our soldiers have been killed by so-called "insider attacks." Lack of understanding and respect for local culture has increased tensions between Afghan forces and our soldiers. Our command requires classes in understanding their culture to mitigate odds of being killed by friendly fire.

It is remarkable that our military requires coursework in understanding culturally diverse colleagues and enemies. Should US civilians be required to understand their culturally diverse fellow citizens before voting and attempting to govern our own country? Is this lack of effort or education part of America's current cultural divide? Do we speak and relate to only those who think like us? Our military is making active efforts to solve their problems. Is this difference just one more example of the demands that we place on our military that we are not willing to make on ourselves?

# CHAPTER ELEVEN
# A JOB FOR ALL AMERICANS: PROXY WITNESS

I recently learned about the job of being a proxy witness from a service member who performs it. As I listened to the job description, I thought that every American should hear this story and perform this job. On second thought, witnessing the effects of war may not be for everyone. Perhaps it should be reserved just for those who believe war is a necessary evil.

The basic skills required are minimal: the ability to speak, listen, and take a few tape measurements.

When the body of a service member returns from war, it has to be received at the morgue. The family has to be received also. Then all that is required is to explain to the family what has happened to their loved one. You might also have to explain why—possibly a little more complicated. Of course, then family members, in their grief, will want to tell you all about what their son, daughter, husband, wife, father, or mother was like until he or she was deployed to war. You will then know well someone you have never met.

After listening to everything the family wants to convey, you will be "personally acquainted" with the deceased. Your job is to leave the family behind and go view the body. Next, you have to measure it. A service member needs a uniform for a proper burial. Uniforms have to be altered to fit bodies that have been altered.

How do you make a uniform for a body with no left leg or right leg or arm? It is probably easier than making one for a body with half a torso missing. What about partial remains? These are questions seldom considered by the average American citizen. If your job, however, is witnessing in the morgue, you have to ask these questions and respond to the answers.

Maybe we citizens should struggle with this basic question: How do I fit a uniform to an altered body? Would that task alter our "uniform" view of the need for war against those who would terrorize us? Some of us would be enraged and want more war.

When we watch the funeral ceremonies on television, it is important to be aware of what has gone on before to make the funeral possible. Someone does serve as our "witness." Most of us have the ability to speak, listen, and take a few tape measurements, but we do not have to witness war and its effects. We are not required to talk about it or even listen. We do not have to personally care for the body of the "fallen."

Wars, seemingly endless and repetitive, are not long enough for every person to take his or her turn performing this job even for one day. Regardless, more exposure to what happens in war might make us think more carefully the next time we consider war.

Ironically, not speaking is what happened to the person who actually performs this job. Five years of meeting families, measuring bodies, and examining the trauma led him to not talk to anyone about it in order "to appear strong." When I first met this person, he was almost unable to speak—only cry, for reasons he did not seem to understand.

Puzzling to him—maybe—but we know why. He has witnessed the unspeakable trauma of wretched dismemberment, disfigurement, and diminishment that none of us has to address. But he has addressed it as "our witness."

## PROFESSIONAL REFLECTION

Dover Air Force Base, America's portal for repatriation, is the front door of our collective living room. The country welcomes into our home the dead bodies of our soldiers who gave their lives for us. Here in this space, our fellow citizens can view and receive the dead body of their relative. Over 20,000 dead from the war in Vietnam were "processed" here. Virtually all deceased soldiers from Afghanistan and Iraq pass through here before being released to their families for a burial in a location of their choice.

Someone has to greet them and meet their families. The soldier I just wrote about does that for each of us. Almost anyone of us is physically qualified to do his work: Just have the ability to speak, listen, and take a few tape measurements. Few of us have the emotional gift or stamina. If we all took turns going to work with him, I suspect it would influence our views about war.

This essay and the next one, "Casualty Service Officer," offer us one opportunity to compare and contrast how the military and civilian society deals with war and death. Islamic militants in Niger killed Sgt. La David Johnson, a member of US Special Forces, in an ambush in October 2017. His body was recovered two days later and flown to Dover Air Force Base for processing. The clarity of Sgt. Johnson's service was compromised by a Congress and administration publicly feuding about the nature of his mission. This ambiguity makes one wonder why American soldiers are dying there.

Myeshia Johnson, his widow, who had known her husband since age six, went to Dover to receive his body. She was apparently advised not to view the body, a suggestion that is often made when a corpse is badly disfigured. In her grief, the inability to personally verify the contents in the casket made mourning her loss all that more difficult. Following a full military funeral, she said, "I'm going to tell (my daughter) how awesome her dad was, and how he was a great father, and how he died a hero."

Her private grieving process is complicated by public officials unable to be civil to one another. A (botched) presidential condolence call allegedly went awry. Her congressperson and the president's chief of staff jumped into the fray. The widow's grieving is compromised by a high-level public "cat fight" between people charged to uphold our constitution and protect our borders. The late Sen. John McCain (R-Ariz.), chairman of the Armed Services Committee, condemned the public dispute over Johnson's death. "We should not be fighting about a brave American who lost his life fighting for his country." AMEN.

Our military knows about ritualized grief and burial. Our public officials appear to be undermining our sense of community.

After each day's work, this soldier who serves as a proxy witness described his one-hour drive to his home. I asked him what the drive is like. He said he cries almost continuously all the way home. It is just part of his service to us.

## CHAPTER TWELVE

# CASUALTY SERVICE OFFICER

"What is your MOS?" I asked one of the routine questions I use.

"Casualty service officer," he replied.

"What does that involve?" I asked, assuming it was not self-evident.

"The Army assigns me to the family of a recently deceased service person, and I stay with that family until everything is taken care of," he said.

"Does that mean you are the one who—"

He interrupted me and said, "Yes, I knock on the door and tell them their loved one is dead."

"Have you had any training?" I asked.

"Some."

"What is it like, breaking the news?"

"The family knows immediately why you are there. They open the door and want to blame someone. Sometimes, they do not want to deal with a Hispanic or black messenger," said this obviously Hispanic-looking black man. Knowing he was both, I asked him how he managed.

Realizing they are distressed and that it is not personal toward him, he surveys the family and determines who the calmest member is. He asks that person to step outside. He tells them that the United States Army and he are prepared to provide the family with everything necessary to deal with this experience. He explains that he will wait as long as necessary for them to consider this information, and he asks them to go back inside to explain to the spouse or father or mother of the deceased what he has said. He asks them to take as long they want to think about it and then to come back to the casualty officer with a decision.

Whatever one thinks about the Army of the United States, they know how to deal with death. And this soldier is one of the more impressive men I have met. Invariably, the family returns for his assistance. Some want to know how he can be helpful with the funeral. Others want to know how much insurance money they will receive. He makes no judgment. He is there to serve.

With little training, I wondered how this man seemed so natural in dealing with complex relationships around the issue of death. He had multiple deployments with some injuries. Still, that did not explain this officer's "street smarts" or intuitive finesse about death. Two other parts of his history were instructive. Recently, he had his own experience with death. He suffered a heart attack and almost died. While he is now recovered with some residual problems, he had personally experienced a near-death experience himself.

Growing up in a large family in a poverty-stricken city taught the officer how to navigate complex relationships. His mother shot his grandfather in front of the children twice. She was not put in jail. His father was the captain of the local police district. This service officer is a man with experience on many levels.

I was privileged to learn more about his work. Being a casualty service officer carries its own set of risks. He meets the body with the family at Dover Air Force Base in Delaware. He is with the family, often for up to six months, arranging for family members' travel, transportation of the body, the viewing, the funeral, the reception, processing the insurance policies, and all the attendant grief work.

He stays with the family until they are, to some degree, at peace with the experience. Some experiences are not peaceful. He recounted one in which the service member had married an Iraqi woman. She and her mother had relocated to the United States. While the husband was redeployed to Iraq, she decided to divorce him. His response: suicide.

It was a complicated situation meeting the body at Dover with the service member's extended family and his wife—the divorce had not been completed. Standing between her and mother as the plane landed, a fight broke out between them. The service member's family blamed the wife for their son's death. Dumbfounded, I asked the casualty officer how he handled that. "I tried to break it up," he said and then rolled up his shirt sleeves to show me all the scratches he had received in this "cat fight."

On the day following our meeting, the casualty service officer was traveling to the cemetery as he had to be there early. The Army protocol mandated that the wife receive the flag after the burial. The Iraqi wife was refusing to accept it. The mother wanted the flag, but protocol required it be given to next of kin. All of this was further complicated because the funerals are routinely videotaped, a copy of which is given to the family. He had "his work cut out for him."

This man and the United States Army perform the burial ritual to perfection. The rifle, the boots, the uniform, the flag and eloquent prayers, the playing of taps and eulogies are a spectacle to behold. They perform a very important service for all of us. If you have never attended a military funeral, it is an experience worth having—even if you do not know the service member who has died.

## PROFESSIONAL REFLECTIONS

As a step in learning how to welcome back a returning soldier, attending a military funeral of any returning soldier is a worthwhile experience. "Sgt. La David Johnson: Killed in Niger, now laid to rest."

https://www.washingtonpost.com/news/checkpoint/wp/2017/10/21/funeral-held-for-sgt-la.

[illegible]

[illegible] comfortable [illegible]

[illegible] limbs [illegible]

[illegible]

# PART IV

# WAR'S EFFECTS ON SOLDIERS

## CHAPTER THIRTEEN

# THE EFFECT OF TRAUMA

The effect of trauma on each soldier is different. As I speak with soldiers, I often wonder what accounts for the variety of responses to trauma. Certainly the degree, intensity, and the frequency of exposure are factors. "How long was your deployment, and how many times were you injured or saw others injured?" are essential questions. While statistical analysis is important, it is not the whole story. In fact, it may not reveal the soldier's story at all.

Some service members seem to sail through the exposure with minimal obvious effect, arguing, "I just did my job." Maybe they hold others responsible for the chaos that they were exposed to or even created. Others have continuing nightmares about a killing even when they found themselves in a "no choice" kill-or-be killed moment. A lot depends on how the soldier experienced the events, and that is often revealed in how the soldier tells his or her story.

The degree of emotional reaction in the individual experiencing the trauma becomes a critical component mediating the traumatic effect. The intensity of this emotional reaction is related to how "connected" an individual is to those involved in the trauma—whether oneself or others. For example, almost everyone would be traumatized by actually seeing his or her best buddy or several buddies killed.

I have come to believe that the trauma effect on soldiers is connected to their relationship to the traumatized person or to the direct trauma experience itself. PTSD, a trauma reaction, is certainly a medical problem like cancer, hypertension, or cardiac disease, but *trauma* has to be approached and understood differently than other medical problems.

The crucible of connections between the trauma and the individuals experiencing and witnessing it is critical. Dave Phillips (2015) in his *New York Times* article entitled "In Unit Stalked by Suicide, Veterans Try to Save One Another," tells a riveting account of the effect of exposure to combat by one Marine unit. He skillfully weaves Marine exposure to trauma, subsequent suffering, and frequent suicide to the nature of their relationship with one another. He reports, "The men of the 2/7 overwhelmingly see a tie between combat and their suicide problem. Not only were all of the men who committed suicide young infantrymen who struggled with experiences of killing and loss, they say, but it is possible to trace one traumatic moment forward and see how those involved are now struggling."

The suicide rate for the Marine combat-exposed unit is fourteen times higher than for Americans in general. One soldier describes being angry about the first few post-deployment suicides he heard about and then was confused after hearing about a few more. Eventually, he became fearful that it was becoming inevitable, like a virus, and that it would kill everyone in the unit. Not only were these Marines traumatized by the initial combat, but they were being retraumatized by each subsequent suicide and ensuing funeral. They began to understand that suicide for them was a post-deployment "combat death."

Listening to their stories or reading Phillips' article, one hears the significance of the relationship connection. Tracking data and keeping statistics in the manner of the US military actually keeps these relationship connections hidden. One report states that deployment in a combat zone is not connected to an increased suicide risk. These studies include in one group all soldiers deployed including the large numbers of support staff not exposed to combat. The studies do not track suicides by individuals in the same unit or who were exposed to the same traumatic experiences. The studies preclude an examination of the relationship between the individual soldiers.

Let me tell you about two soldiers I recently worked with who further illustrate the importance of relationship. Later, I will report on what the soldiers are suggesting as a way to possibly remedy this problem.

Sgt. Jones has had several deployments to Iraq and Afghanistan. He was a squad leader responsible for a number of other service members. Exposed to mortars, artillery, machine guns, RPGs, and IEDs, he suffered only a few shrapnel wounds. He was "constantly at risk," with "no front line," and where "everything was fair game." He said he grew weary of bagging body parts of comrades to be sorted out later by others. Convinced he would not "get out alive," he gained comfort by focusing "on effectiveness not safety." Accepting the fact that he "was already dead" gave him "the relief to care for others."

Now home, this soldier is reunited with his family, and he cannot figure out "how to come back to life or how to be alive." He feels numb, empty, without joy as he tries "to play the part" of father and husband. A good soldier—whose relationships were so traumatized—he has lost the ability to relate to himself and to others. He is working on "remembering his colleagues." He knows he cannot change what happened, but he hopes he can remember them for who they were and not for what happened to them.

Sgt. Miller has had multiple deployments to Iraq and Afghanistan as well. He is a mortician and is responsible for finding, collecting, and putting together human remains. He believes he is in good health and has only minor complaints. While deployed, he is rarely if ever exposed to combat fire. He works with human remains on a daily basis. He describes the "smell as unique" but believes he has "the stomach" for the work. He knows most of the morticians in the military and all those who have committed suicide. He believes that his military occupational specialty has the highest rate of suicide of any job category.

He strongly advises colleagues to avoid anything that connects them personally to the human remains with which they work. He does not "want to develop any emotional relationship to the remains." He believes he is doing his job for surviving family members so they can "pay their respects in the context of their beliefs." He describes himself "as almost never having a bad day."

The subject of trauma is of course more complicated than just the stories of Sgt. Jones, Sgt. Miller, and those mentioned in the Phillips' article. However, their stories do illustrate the importance of one's relationship to trauma and to the person traumatized.

The members of the Marine unit, as described by Phillips, learned to depend on one another to survive in combat. Now, they have banded together using new software and social media "to create a quick response system that allows them to track, monitor, and intervene with some of their most troubled comrades" at risk for post-combat death.

They have organized their post-combat relationships through social media with the same altruism as their combat relationships. They just might have something there—depending on relationships—that gives them a way to reduce these post-combat deaths. How can we best support them in their efforts to help each other?

## PROFESSIONAL REFLECTIONS

**These soldiers are there by choice in our place. If you do not think they should be there, then advocate for stopping wars. If you agree with them standing in your place, then you owe them more than a "thank you for your service." Listen to how a soldier tells his or her story. How the story is told is a key to understanding their relationship to trauma and to the traumatized person.**

Citizens may not have direct responsibility for combat trauma, but citizens do have a responsibility to help eliminate or reduce post-deployment suffering. The Marine combat unit as featured in the Phillips article describes one way to help. They have devised a social media response system to prevent post-combat deaths. Making a relationship with a soldier and being willing to listen to the suffering of soldiers is an important first step.

Each of us can contribute. Sgt. Miller's job was to collect bodies so that surviving family members could "pay their respects in the context of their beliefs." He made it possible for family members to bury their dead. Sgt. Jones, a hero, returning alive, has forgotten how to live. Numb, and joyless, he is temporarily lacking the ability to be a father or a spouse. He needs a mentor, an important relationship, or a group in which to learn about relationships. No effort is too small. The remediation could begin over coffee, the newspaper, at church, the bowling alley, little league baseball, soccer practice, at the grocery store, or in the middle of the night—any time where small acts of kindness are possible. When you see him, try to get to know him. If at first you don't succeed, try again.

## CHAPTER FOURTEEN

# "SOMETHING AWFUL HAD TO HAPPEN TO GET US HELP!"

Many of us watched the Memorial Day tribute to the Unknown Soldier. I believe President Obama when he says we should honor the dead by providing service to the living. A good idea.

Earlier, the Secretary of Veterans Affairs said they were working to provide "timely service to veterans." Another good idea. Later, they acknowledged that 24,000 veterans had been improperly evaluated for traumatic brain injury, and they would all be reevaluated. At the Memorial Day Concert on the Washington Mall, celebrities lauded the service of veterans from all wars. The message was, "We care; if you need help, someone is available. Dial this number and press option 1." Awkward, but I believe these platitudes were sincerely stated.

Yet, we know there is another side of this story. So much war, so little peace for both the nation and for individuals.

A servicewoman recently came for an initial appointment. Her story was all too familiar. But the precipitating event for the appointment was unusual. Her history suggested she was quite resourceful and resilient. As a teenage mother, she managed to finish high school then join the Army, finish college, and work on a master's degree. Along the way, she found time to raise a second child.

Seven years before this initial visit, she had been raped while in the Army. This soldier had experienced trauma and, while deployed, witnessed significant atrocities. Fearing the "consequences of reporting," she experienced the effects of the rape but never sought treatment nor reported the events. She perceived that reporting in the military meant she would be ostracized, marginalized, and her career would be over. She claimed to have witnessed that happening to other soldiers on multiple occasions.

She believed that once a soldier seeks mental health treatment, a code is broken. The soldier can expect an administrative or medical discharge or poor assignments. Her husband, a veteran, shared her view in not getting treatment for abuse or combat-related trauma while on active duty.

But now as a veteran it was clear to both of them that he needed help for his depression, irritability, and hypervigilance—in essence, he needed help for his combat-related PTSD. They waited for an inpatient-based program rather than an outpatient program. Month after month, they were told that no beds were available.

As symptoms increased, marital conflict and tension increased. Her husband chose to commemorate an anniversary of the combat death of a good friend with a visit to a local bar. Left with sleepless children, she angrily took them to the car and drove them around the block, trying to get them to fall asleep.

When her husband returned home, intoxicated, he perceived that she had abandoned him. An angry confrontation ensued. Unfortunately, they are both authorized to carry concealed weapons. She thought putting her hand on her weapon would bring him to his senses. Instead, he thought he was going to be killed and attacked her. She escaped. Police arrived. He was taken away. She reported the incident. A hospital-based program was available for him the next morning.

"Something bad had to happen to get us help," she says.

So much war, so little peace—both for the nation and for our veterans. Need it be this way so often?

## PROFESSIONAL REFLECTIONS

This essay presents many of the problems soldiers and veterans confront: sexual trauma, combat trauma, availability of guns, alcohol use, marriage to one another, and problems in the availability of treatment. Among Veterans who use VA health care, about 23 percent of women reported sexual assault while serving in the military. According to the US Department of Veteran Affairs, the total number of vets reporting military sexual trauma represent more male service members than female because there are so many more men in the service.

This couple initially worried more about potential stigma for their conditions than getting help. It took them a long time to realize they could not change what other people thought. They could reduce their own mental health problems from getting in the way of performing their own jobs and living their own lives. Getting mental health service can be complicated. All service members deployed in recent wars are potentially eligible for service-connected disease treatment and disability compensation. The Associated Press reports that about 45 percent of post 9/11 veterans will seek disability claims. This is a large group of individuals for the VA to evaluate and treat. A National Bureau of Economic Research paper states that signing up for services is "long, cumbersome, inefficient and paperwork-intensive."

The incidence of PTSD, TBI, and chronic depression among soldiers is higher than for the civilian population. Studies vary but suffice to say, there are hundreds of thousands of soldiers in each category. Modern medicine and streamlined trauma services lead to fewer combat deaths but more soldiers surviving with combat physical and mental health injury. In WWII, there were two injuries per soldier killed. In Vietnam, there were 2.6 injuries per soldier killed; and in Iraq, there have been sixteen injuries per soldier killed. More soldiers are surviving with scars requiring treatment.

Civilian Medicare is funded predictably, like Social Security, from an ongoing trust fund. Military health care is unpredictably funded from the US budget each year and is subjected regularly to unpredictable political winds. By 2020, the price of treating Iraq and Afghanistan veterans alone could be more than $8 billion annually, according to the CBO.

In "Battleland: Military Intelligence for the Rest of Us," Mark Thompson (2012) reported that the cost to the VA of treating an individual case of PTSD in the first year is $8,300; TBI is $11,700; or both are about $20,000. The cost is about five times the cost of treating vets with neither diagnosis. Cost of treating their families is additional, as is the cost of divorce, which is higher in these families. The difficulty in predicting the ongoing incidence of these conditions makes financial and medical planning quite complicated.

The Veterans Administration, the second largest agency in the United States government, continues to make progress in the treatment of these conditions according to the National Center for PTSD.

## CHAPTER FIFTEEN

# PERFECT SOLUTION OR PERFECT STORM?

Substantially more wounded soldiers survive their injuries in this war than in prior wars. The military is attempting to provide the best care possible for these survivors. A soldier wounded in Afghanistan can expect to be back in a hospital in Germany within hours. These "volunteer" soldiers are more physically and mentally traumatized than the "draftees" of other wars. The Veterans Administration is systematically hiring medical staff to deal with the increasing numbers of disabled casualties. Seamless acute and chronic care is an appropriate societal goal for these heroes.

I work to provide "telepsychiatric services" to military bases that are short staffed of mental health providers. Ideally, our service can flexibly adapt to shortages wherever they occur. Recently, a survivor came to me for a medication renewal. His psychiatrist had diagnosed him with PTSD but was moving and could no longer provide care for this survivor. The patient said he just needed some more antidepressant and sleep medication. As with all new patients, I insisted he tell me his history.

He knew in high school that he wanted to be a medic. After graduation, he enlisted and went through all the training. Deployed in Iraq and later Afghanistan, he was proud of his service. He met his wife while in training; they lived together for over a year and then were married. She was waiting for him after he returned from his first deployment.

His second deployment was more traumatic. There were long days of flying out to pick up wounded or dead soldiers, and landing a helicopter on a mountainside was extremely difficult. At about fifty feet, the rotary blades cause a "dust up," which means the pilot has to land blind. Day after day, the work became traumatizing. He sought behavioral health treatment while deployed and was started on medication for his depression and sleep difficulties, all while continuing his work.

One week before his long anticipated reconnection with his wife, she contacted him, informing him that she was no longer living in their home. When he arrived there, he found it "trashed" with no sign of his wife. Months later, his search located her in a nearby town, pregnant and living with another man. Like many returning service members, he turned to alcohol for consolation.

One night, he and a colleague were comparing pistols. He owned a very small one. After a few drinks, they went "bar hopping." While drinking at the bar his cell phone rang and, unfortunately, he reached in the wrong pocket and pulled out the small pistol. Observed by the bouncer, he was arrested. An enlightened Army personnel member noted that his problem was an alcohol and behavioral-health one and not a planned illegal act. The soldier was placed in a substance abuse treatment facility for one month. He was discharged with PTSD and continued to struggle with depression and substance abuse. Having no support from his spouse, he attempted to reconnect with his family with whom he maintained close emotional ties. Because of his "crime," he was not allowed to travel.

As time passed, he began to think that the Army was monitoring his behavior. Cars passing his house seemed to be observing him. He bought a police scanner to monitor the traffic. He believed phone calls from his parents were really Army personnel in disguise. Luckily, Army medical staff recognized his psychosis and he was hospitalized. One month of successful hospital treatment led to a discharge.

He resolved to divorce his estranged wife as she gave birth to the other man's child. State law mandates that the child is legally his because he is married to the child's mother. The law does not recognize the physical separation at conception. His wife refused to complete paperwork to allow the divorce and for proper recording of the paternity of the child. His psychosis returned, and he was rehospitalized. Successful treatment, followed by long-term outpatient psychotherapy, resolved his psychosis.

Three hospitalizations and continuing symptoms of PTSD led to a medical determination that he should be honorably discharged from the military. He was referred to the Warrior Transition Unit, recently devised to streamline medical treatment and the transition to civilian life.

One of the symptoms of PTSD is a "sense of a foreshortened future" (e.g., the person does not expect to have a career, marriage, children, or a normal life span). This soldier's experience endorses that symptom. It raises the question, however: Is that PTSD or good reality testing?

What to say! This soldier is a previously motivated, highly competent medic anticipating college and a career in medicine. Now in his early twenties with three mental-health hospitalizations and major medical problems, he has received all the proper treatment for his conditions. It would be hard to criticize his medical treatment.

His wife is gone. His anticipated career may be gone. He provided good service *to* the Army. He was given good service *by* the Army. Undoubtedly, he will be financially compensated for his disability.

For this warrior and our country, is this a perfect solution or a perfect storm?

## PROFESSIONAL REFLECTIONS

I am not certain there is anything to add to this soldier's story and concluding question. Perhaps it means that we civilians just need to think about its implications.

## CHAPTER SIXTEEN

# I MET WITH A GUY TODAY WHO . . .

I met with a guy today who said he was having a very bad day. I have seen this soldier many times over the past year. He has improved reasonably well, so I was puzzled at how bad he was feeling. He and I had been working for months on his PTSD.

"Today is the tenth anniversary of the day my young medic died," he began. "I have to call his parents. They know the call is coming from me and from several others who always remember. They anticipate the call for days ahead with all the anxiety and depression and sadness that surround it. Sometimes, I think it's better not to call, to cause them all that pain, but I can't fail to call. I can't fail to remember him.

"Americans don't understand what it's like for parents to get their last letter, their last phone call, the last photograph, and know that they have had their last conversation with their son or daughter. Almost worse is not knowing *when* that might be. Then the child is gone and the parents just have our phone calls—once a year. They are appreciative, but we are no substitute.

"He was a young kid, always smiling. He didn't like others being in a bad mood, so he was always trying to cheer up everyone else. He was a medic for fifty men. Every Tuesday morning, he would wake us up for our antimalarial pills. He'd make us take them. If we were in a bad mood yelling, 'Get away from me,' he'd pick a fight, take off his shirt and start fighting, and then break down laughing and smiling in a comical way. 'Aha, I got you to laugh,' he'd say.

"He truly believed he was put on this earth to make us happy.

"When he died, the trigger guys, the snipers—the ones who are trained to kill the bad guys—went to our commander. With tears in their eyes, they asked the commander, 'We are supposed to die; he is supposed to care for us; how can this happen?' They loved him so much. Now, I think, he is in heaven trying to make angels happy."

Without changing pace, and almost as if he were not changing the subject, the soldier began talking about how angry he was with his eighteen-year-old son.

"I am at my wits' end with him. I try to correct his behavior. If I get physical, he says I cannot do that because it is child abuse, and he will call the Department of Social Services." He asked, "If he runs away, can I grab him and bring him home? No, because I cannot cause bodily harm or injury to him. When I catch him in a lie, he accuses me of something. Even his friend who witnessed his behavior said to him, 'Do you ever listen to your parents?' He is supposed to take medication, but I never know if he is taking it or not. He goes all over town with his friends. We never know exactly where he is."

The soldier has friends throughout the community who he has asked regularly to report his son's behavior to him. Plus, he put a secret tracking device on his son's phone so he can monitor his whereabouts.

This soldier has given me a lot to think about. I see that somehow he has connected emotionally his frustration with the death of his medic to his perceived failure as a parent. He now sees himself as helpless in both situations, and it has united his anger in each. If I were to say that directly to him, that might sound too confrontational and maybe offensive. I can only imagine his response would be something like, "Well, doc, how would you feel if your best colleague were killed and now your son will not obey you?"

I asked him how in fact his son is doing in school and whether he has ever been really irresponsible. He acknowledged that his son does well in school, does not take drugs, has never committed a crime, has a good peer group, and never goes to "bad areas of the community." He further added that his son does well away from him and that he, himself, seems to do better at work away from his son.

It is obvious to me that this soldier has his PTSD symptoms overly focused on his son's behavior. In combination—his hyperalertness, hypervigilance, worry and preoccupation, guilt, trying to make amends—are all focused on his son, who happens to not be too much younger than his medic.

Trying to reduce the intensity of the emotional focus, I said, "You are working too hard at making your son behave!"

"Everyone tells me that," he responded.

"So, why not take the advice," I suggested. As he pondered, I added, "Furthermore I have one more suggestion that you may think is a crazy idea."

"I can handle it," he said.

"You are a very compassionate, concerned, connected human being who really cares about others. Your son does not see that side of you, nor understand it. I think your relationship with him would benefit by seeing that side of you.

"Will you go home and tell your son all that you have told me today about the loss of your young medic, and the impact it has had on you, and how it makes you suffer?"

"Sure, I can do that," he said, very quickly.

Eager for the next appointment, I remain troubled by the lack of reflection in his response. Had he accepted my "crazy" suggestion because he is a "good soldier" following orders? Does he really see the connection between his anger and helplessness in both circumstances? Will his son make the connection? Do they need to understand it or will just presenting a different side of him to his son make a sufficient impact on their relationship?

I don't know the answer. I do know that war can wreak havoc on parenting.

## PROFESSIONAL REFLECTIONS

This soldier's story illustrates how his emotional response to military and civilian life can overlap. Anger, irritability, and emotional numbing and withdrawal are common. Soldiers are reluctant to discuss their military trauma, believing they will traumatize family members. There are cases in which spouses and children are traumatized just by living with a family member with PTSD.

The veteran's inability to feel emotionally close and his reluctance to disclose trauma-related memories complicates family life. This reluctance and inability creates friction and distance among family members. Children may feel uncared for by a parent appearing disinterested. Adolescents may be overly reactive to a hypervigilant parent or conversely overidentify with them and act in the same manner. Sleeping spouses may be misidentified as "the enemy" as a soldier is awakened by a traumatic nightmare.

Soldiers with PTSD divorce at twice the rate in first marriages as soldiers without it and are three times as likely to divorce more than once. Child abuse in these families is increased. The burden assumed by spouses in these families is substantial both objectively and subjectively. According to the National Center for PTSD, families need to understand that they are living with someone whose mind has been altered by his/her combat experience.

Family education about PTSD is critical. Spouses and children need to understand that no matter how personally directed, the trauma symptoms are not about them. Individual therapy followed by couples and family therapy can be very helpful. The grief work needed by traumatized veterans is a family matter—one that should be a national priority.

I hope this soldier and his son were able to have this conversation about the impact of the war on their relationship.

## CHAPTER SEVENTEEN

# CHOICES: 2016

"No Boots on the Ground," "No Fly Zones," "Safe Zones on the Ground," "Carpet Bombing," "Make the Sand Glow!" "Special Ops," "Strategic Air Campaign," "Strategically Grounded Diplomatic Initiatives."

These statements are among the various choices offered to voters by current political candidates regarding combating terrorism. Which option do you prefer? What if you really had to choose to fight terrorism, or worse yet, were forced to do so! What options would you choose?

Would you choose one of these offered by our politicians? Would you actually do the fighting, or would you choose not to fight? Would you personally send someone to do the fighting for you? Whether we realize it or not, we have sent someone else to war in our place and continue to do so. On this issue, our democratic society has spoken and will get an opportunity to do so again in upcoming elections.

Given the terrorism that has occurred in Paris and California recently, it is understandable that some of us are fearful. These popular political solutions trivialize the enormity of the problem of fighting terrorism or protecting refugees of terrorism. These are the choices our politicians offer. Does anyone really know which answer is correct?

I have the privilege of asking soldiers on a regular basis about these choices. Speaking to them and being sensitive to what may be behind their point of view, it is hard to know how much questioning is too much. Almost universally, they say, "You do not really want to know."

Often, I respond, "What is it that you think we do not want to know?" They usually don't want to tell. "No Boots on the Ground" in fact involves "Special Ops"—people who put themselves in very dangerous places, landing aircraft in dirt fields with no airstrip, working long hours under intense and treacherous conditions until soldiers say, "Your body forgets how to fall asleep."

Taking prisoners can be just the beginning of the problems. Holding them behind temporary fences can lead to a breakdown in civilized behavior within those fences. They may try to kill one another; escorting them for "bathroom breaks" often requires that the soldier dress in a full suit of protective armor. Soldiers in these situations experience hypervigilance as "normal." Afterward, many return unable or unwilling to share their experiences with their family. Some come to see a psychiatrist saying, "Doc, I am fine, but I am losing my family!" They are unable to talk about these extreme situations, especially with those who have not experienced it.

Recently, I saw a soldier who had participated in four deployments, all in locations we associate with "harm's way." This particular soldier was deployed on the original search for weapons of mass destruction. I asked if he suffered any physical injury in that or the subsequent three deployments. "No physical injuries," he said. "But, I am losing my family. I fight with them over the silliest of things and do not even say hello when I come home from work." Then he spends the rest of the night on his computer until it is time to go to sleep and have nightmares. Puzzled, I had to ask again, "Were you physically injured or rendered unconscious?"

"I was lucky," he said, "no physical injuries."

"No exposure to combat?" I asked.

"Well, my vehicle was bombed and rolled over ten times," he admitted. He went on, "I was in several direct-fire gun battles. I was shelled by mortars. A number of my friends died. I took the life of many people. People died two feet in front of me.

"I resigned myself to dying. If it comes, it comes. I did what I was told to do, what my country ordered me to do. It was not heroic. I was not the kind of man I wanted to be. What we did was a waste of time implementing a political agenda. There were no weapons of mass destruction. While I was deployed, one of my family members committed suicide.

"I cannot describe what actually happened. If you really want to know, go deploy. People who want to volunteer to fight are crazy. I know if you do, you will never be the same. I will never be the same as I was. I try to drown myself in alcohol, but that doesn't work. And yet, I was not physically injured."

Struggling to make a connection through all this, I asked if the movie *American Sniper* captured what he was talking about. "No," he said, "the combat scenes seem contrived" and not real to him. "Maybe the D-Day invasion in *Saving Private Ryan* comes closer," he said.

What we are told by politicians and what our servicemen and women are experiencing are starkly different realities. What choices are we making? Are we even aware we are making these choices?

Shouldn't we remember what our deepest belief is as human beings and embed that belief into our choices?

## PROFESSIONAL REFLECTIONS

I realize I am arguing for civilians to be involved in talking with soldiers, and this essay describes soldiers not wanting to talk with civilians. Yet, the conversation about death and dying cannot be left at an impasse. Continuing silence is a disservice to those who have served and to those who have died. We honor their service by knowing what they did and remembering their service.

By listening and hearing, we will enhance our understanding of war and the wisdom we will need in deciding about starting the "next" war. I am describing what soldiers do not want to share and we have to find a way to listen. The choices framed by politicians seem like bland jargon: "No Boots on the Ground" and "Strategically Grounded Diplomatic Initiatives." The choice executed by this soldier alleges a life-changing experience: "I will never be the same as I was. I was not the kind of man I want to be."

In addition to behaving in a personally unacceptable manner, he believes his country misled him. Rather than making the country safer, he feels he was just implementing a political agenda. He experienced moral injury not physical injury. His inability to emotionally metabolize what he saw and experienced and discuss is driving his family away from him. He must find a way to share his story. He has returned from a universe of behavior so unlike ours that he cannot find an acceptable place for himself in our more conventional life.

What politicians proclaim and what soldiers experience are starkly different realities. They both represent us civilians. What do we want them to do on our behalf? In our recent times, in response to their experience of life-changing violence, schoolchildren are saying, "Enough is enough." Shouldn't we remember what our deepest belief is as human beings and embed that belief into our decisions about war?

## CHAPTER EIGHTEEN

# THE SOLUTION IS MORE MORAL THAN MEDICAL

Colleagues ask me what I do. When I answer, they frequently respond, "See a lot of PTSD, I guess." "Well, yes, but many service members suffer from 'plain old depression,' " I say. These individuals often feel profoundly lonely in a crowd and utterly helpless and hopeless. Their disorders differ by duration and timing of the symptoms and also their cause.

The incidence of depression in the world has increased substantially each decade in the past 100 years. Epidemiologists speculate about the cause. A November 2013 article in the journal *PLOS Medicine* (Public Library of Science, a journal of peer-reviewed, open-access research articles) reported a worldwide map of depression that showed the highest incidence of reported depression in the world was in Afghanistan, the Palestinian Territories, and North Africa as well as Eritrea and Rwanda. It does not take much imagination to realize what these places have in common: war and a lot of combat.

A soldier who witnesses many traumatized and dead bodies can experience depression. When soldiers regret what they have seen and done, even though they signed up to do it—that can also cause depression. Having trouble controlling your anger until it becomes overwhelming can also be a factor. Killing someone in the heat of battle, no matter how justified in the moment, can be experienced quite differently by the soldier when back home in the United States in the "comfort" of one's family.

Most experience the common symptoms of depression—problems with mood; feeling down, up and down, or just empty. Many suffer difficulty falling asleep or staying asleep or waking up too early. There may be problems with appetite or weight. Often, individuals have somatic complaints, pain or dysfunction in one's body. Somatic symptoms are more difficult to treat, but the pharmaceutical industry created one drug specifically designed for somatic symptoms as well as created drugs for most of the other symptoms. There is always "talking." Good psychotherapy may work as well as the drugs.

The one symptom that is more difficult is anhedonia: NO JOY IN LIFE. In my decades of private practice, I have seen people complaining of mostly all the symptoms mentioned above. Not often do I see someone who experiences no pleasure in living.

Recently, I was confronted with this problem more forcefully than ever. A young female medic appeared for an appointment. Deployed three times, her depression began after the second deployment. Initially, it went away slowly. After the third deployment, the depression did not leave her. She had tried a number of antidepressants without success. It was not immediately clear if she self-prescribed or persuaded someone else to prescribe for her. Currently, she was on an appropriate but insufficient amount of a medication and said, "I have anhedonia." I guess she wanted to sound rather professional, using a technical term, rather than seem to be a suffering patient who had no joy. She wanted a medication to solve this problem and had a list of medication possibilities.

For the past one and one-half years, she thought daily of shooting herself. "Don't worry," she said, "if I decide to kill myself, there is nothing you can do to stop me." And then she cited all the ways she could obtain a gun and ammunition in this state or another. Her intentions were believable and serious.

Needing to get more information, I asked a lot of questions. Her appetite and weight were fine. She could fall asleep for three to five hours and feel rested. She had adequate energy working long hours taking care of others. But she was clearly not the person she had been before her deployments. There was nothing from which she gathered either satisfaction or enjoyment. She exercised but got no satisfaction from it. She hiked but no longer enjoyed being outdoors. Her family life was stable but emotionally distant. The last thing she had enjoyed was her deployment in which she worked with a very sophisticated medical team taking care of wounded and dying soldiers. She had a list of reasons: "I saw the best and the worst. I would return to work with those soldiers at a moment's notice. I felt more connected to people than ever in my life. The quality of the work was exceptional. It was an expensively satisfying experience because it came at a great emotional price.

"It was not free," she surmised.

I asked if she had talked to anyone else about her depression. "Yes," she said, "I went to my commander." "And?" I asked. "He told me 'to get over it or get out of the Army.' " Stigma persists. She followed with, "I currently work as a medic in the most toxic environment imaginable, much worse than being deployed."

"How about your clergy?" I asked. She'd had a number of meetings with the chaplain but felt he listened without really trying to understand.

Speaking as if I had not heard, she said, "I did not consent to being born." I thought it was one of the most astonishing statements a patient ever uttered. Was she saying, "I am alive against my own wishes? I did not want to be born. Life is not a gift."

Had she no spiritual life? Did Pentecost make no sense? Where was her faith? Did she not accept God's acceptance of her? Clearly, she was authorizing her right to take her own life.

That astonishing comment coupled with "deployment comes at a price" led me to say, "What makes you think your problem is medical? I think it might be more a moral one." She had wondered the same thing.

"Why did you survive and so many others did not?" I asked.

"I did not make any mistakes," she responded. Is that what life is all about—not **a gift** but rather not making any mistakes?

We have different perspectives! But she is down a foxhole into which I am having a hard time reaching her.

"What if I do not make another appointment?" she said. I thought the moral rather than medical approach was pertinent and I said, "I will come after you." She deserves no less.

## PROFESSIONAL REFLECTIONS

Happiness and joy in life can be elusive. The United States Declaration of Independence declares the right to pursue happiness, not be happy. Soldiers and civilians pursue it in different ways. This medic appeared happy or at least happier while serving her country as part of an efficient and effective medical team in combat. She "currently works as a medic in the most toxic environment imaginable, much worse than being deployed." Her commander is overtly hostile to mental health problems and lacks compassion. Her current unit and her role in it are quite different from the one in which she deployed.

Individuals in combat units protect one another. The mutual trust intertwined with responsibility for one another provides confidence and self-assurance. They are like angels watching over one another. Doing a job well, especially one that saves lives, is inspiring. When the job involves continuous exposure to trauma, it chips away at one's humanity. Soldiers speak of dying in war while continuing to live. Guilt over surviving when a colleague dies can lead to emotional distance and withdrawal from relationships. The adrenaline high that is experienced in the heat of battle can obscure this personal loss of humanity. The relatively slower pace of stateside service leaves more time for contemplation.

I think this soldier had difficultly processing what she saw and did during deployment. The deployment was defining too much of who she was. She had difficulty reclaiming a better sense of herself and grieving about what she saw. The absence of close friends, family, and an unsympathetic command officer made reconstructing who she was more complicated. She needs to find and to make use of a social environment as effective and trusting as was her combat unit. America owes to this soldier an environment in which to regain her humanity.

# PART V

# WAR'S EFFECT ON CIVILIANS

CHAPTER NINETEEN

# CREATING LEISURE SPACE WITH COLLEAGUES

We are a large group of mental health providers who provide telehealth services to soldiers around the country. We examine and treat soldiers across vast geographic distance over closed circuit television. We are psychiatrists, psychologists, social workers, physical therapists, registered nurses, language specialists, and a few other medical specialists. If asked, most of us might be opposed to war as a method of solving conflict. Yet, we all seem drawn to the task of providing care for injured soldiers.

Our diverse group is composed of men and women, old and young, African American, Caucasian, Asian American, Native American, Anglo European, Caribbean, Pakistani, Indian, Jewish, Catholic, Protestant, Muslim, and Hindu.

The common goal of treating servicemen and women has created a certain emotional bond among us. We all understand that a soldier's first duty is to care for his or her buddy. Caring for the other ensures the safety of the unit and that others will look after you. One among our evolving problems while taking care of soldiers is the problem of how to take care of ourselves. That necessity is not very obvious at first and certainly on the surface does not seem as important. It is the antithesis of what soldiers do. They take care of themselves by taking care of their buddies. What happens to the mental health providers as they care for others, and what should they do about it?

We find ourselves "chatting" a lot. Hospitality at Walter Reed is infectious. The Army has made comforting others a first-order mandate in recent years. Soldiers are unfailingly polite and courteous. It is easy to follow their example.

Among ourselves, we often talk about the type of "presenting problems" of soldiers. Those less experienced providers ask the more experienced ones about medications, indications, side effects, and what type of treatments are most effective. When homicidal or suicidal situations arise, we often seek second and third opinions about the most appropriate intervention.

Smaller groups of the larger whole of mental health providers began to meet to have lunch or to discuss "clinical issues." While at Walter Reed, it was an "experience" to eat together in the cafeteria with all the service members. The Army protocol and the unfailing hospitality were comforting. The depth and breadth of the soldiers' physical trauma in the cafeteria was a constant reminder of the reason for our work. It was inspiring to watch soldiers with multiple amputations manage the cafeteria lines, the crowded rooms, the tables to feed themselves while having an enjoyable conversation with colleagues.

BRAC, the Base Closure and Realignment Commission, changed all of that for us. We have been temporarily moved to a downtown high-rise building secured by the Army. The small military presence is still there but attenuated in intensity. We no longer have a cafeteria with service members. A smaller group of us has created, rather, a lunchroom environment.

Our conversations in our "new lunchroom" have changed. Previously, we talked about the usual things: politics, family, courtship, and marriage. Older married providers advised younger singles about dating. On Valentine's Day, we went overboard with advice.

We have had a chance to discuss and compare notes and reading material on war. Some of us served in prior wars. Some of us grew up with relatives who fought in war. As mental health workers, we noted how much easier it was to fight in wars when the other was "hated or foreign." Fighting an insurgency is far more complicated. The diversity of our group highlights that issue. Those of us born in America listen carefully as our Pakistani and Indian colleagues discuss their views on Afghanistan and the tense relationship between their own two countries.

The end points of many days are mundane. A problem is presented as routine, one heard many times, and there is a standard solution. The patient is understood, and the provider knows what to do. These transactions occur over and over in a sort of routine way throughout the day for many of us. Yet recently, our conversation has changed again. Some of us noted a tension at the end of each clinical session. At the close of the day, some clinicians said they were exhausted: not physically but emotionally.

There are days when these encounters bring one face to face with ideas, events, and action one has never seen or possibly never heard about: Soldiers anguishing over the unintentional killing of children; colleagues disintegrated by IEDs, essentially unseen landmines; soldiers uncovering mass gravesites and having continuing nightmares; soldiers with survivor guilt; soldiers blamed by relatives for the death of their loved one.

In general, we are an experienced group. One senior member volunteered that recently he has been having great difficulty getting out of bed in the morning to come to work. One provider noted that he is less interested in socializing with others. A second noted that he is no longer interested in "routine problems" of patients and has a hard time dealing with the "mundane" conflicts of others. Another provider reports that in social situations she has been verbally attacked by others for allegedly "supporting the war effort."

The caring for others is having its effects. Interestingly, we are now after months and months of talking to traumatized soldiers becoming aware of its effect on us. Creating this leisure space—the "lunchroom"—has allowed us the opportunity to talk among ourselves. Talking with others is certainly helpful. We advocate it for soldiers. Sharing pain of trauma seems to make it a little more tolerable, but its long-term effects remain troubling.

One of the providers thinks the soldiers need a more comprehensive framework to understand their experiences. He believes "a job well done" professed by the soldiers is not sufficient to manage the effects of killing. He is working on a guideline to help them understand their guilt and by implication find a way to forgive themselves. What a thought! Here we are a nation sending out young men to kill the enemy and now looking for ways in which they can forgive themselves for what we asked them to do. I hope he works it out. If he is successful, maybe it will be something for our nation to "chew on" during its leisure time. Forgive ourselves before we do this again.

## PROFESSIONAL REFLECTIONS

Our group of professional mental health providers was almost as diverse as is America. Our cultural, political, ethnic, racial, and religious differences were easily put aside by our desire to work cooperatively with and provide care for our servicemen and women. This is an example of what America can do for itself—find a way out of its tribalism by service for a common good. The rights we all enjoy as citizens come with certain responsibilities.

The selective service, our common draft, is over. We still register eighteen-year-olds but with almost no expectation that they would serve in the military. Our country is now protected by a professional volunteer force. We could, however, expect everyone to provide some national service in return for our rights as citizens.

During the war in Vietnam, nightly we witnessed on television the trauma of war. Our country became so distressed by the carnage that citizens in effect brought a halt to the war by protesting it. Similar episodic carnage occurs in our civilian life at Pulse Orlando nightclub, Virginia Tech in Blacksburg, Sandy Hook Elementary School, Luby's Cafeteria in Killeen, Texas, Columbine High School, and most recently at the Marjory Stoneman Douglas High School in Parkland, Florida, in Dayton, Ohio and El Paso, Texas. and Tree of Life Synagogue, Pittsburgh, Emanuel African Methodist Episcopal Church in Charleston SC, and the travesty of immigration treatment on the Southern border. Commentators warn us not to look at the television footage as it might be too traumatic even if seen by remote bystanders.

Civilians comfort one another after these episodic civilian tragedies. Survivors of Sandy Hook in Connecticut journey to Parkland, Florida, to minister to the survivors of the Marjory Stoneman Douglas killings; student to student, teacher to teacher, and student and teacher together band together in order that the students might reenter the school. Our nation struggles to find a way to work for the common good.

But soldiers and first responders manage carnage each day so that we do not have to do so. They provide vicarious service for us. They experience not only physical trauma but also moral trauma from their work. Moral trauma can lead to estrangement from one's self or one another. As soldiers try to reenter civilian society, we owe a "listening ear" to them just as effectively as we respond to grief of our fellow civilians. Soldiers witness for us. Much of America's grief remains within our soldiers, and we owe it to them to find a way to share in their service.

## CHAPTER TWENTY

# "IT GOES BOTH WAYS"

In my decades as a psychiatrist, I've seen many kinds of patients; only in recent years, though, have I worked with soldiers.

I see them through an organization that offers patients long-distance care. I originally took this job for financial reasons (in 2010, after the start of the economic downturn of 2008), but I quickly discovered its unique rewards.

Early on, for instance, as I stood waiting for an elevator, a quadriplegic soldier maneuvered his electric wheelchair alongside me. When the doors opened, he looked up and said, "After you, sir." That's not a memory that fades.

Unfortunately, I also discovered the job's difficulties. At times, despite my admiration for the soldiers' heroism and bravery, I've found it hard to hear so many stories of death, loss, and grief.

Also, commuting to work has become progressively more arduous. Initially, I worked at Walter Reed, but our telehealth group has grown so much that we've had to move twice. These days, in place of my original twenty-minute commute, I drive to the subway parking lot, walk to the Metro, take a forty-five-minute ride, then walk fifteen minutes underground to my new workplace.

Finally, since our building is controled by the Department of Defense, we're subject to rigorous security requirements. No one can enter or exit the building or offices without the requisite badges and whistles, and the arrangements are complex and ever-changing—passes expire, codes change, bureaucracy is ever-present.

At times, this work's psychological and logistical stresses have made me wonder, How can I continue? and ask myself whether I should stop out of self-preservation. All of this brings me to recent events.

Less than twenty-four hours before the start of a telepsychiatry session, I suffered a personal trauma of my own: the loss of a beloved family member. Despite my grief, though, I never considered canceling the session; as always, it seemed to me that the soldier's need for support outweighed mine.

The next morning, I drove to the Metro, boarded the subway, and walked to work as always. As I reached the building entrance, I suffered a horrifying realization: I had left behind all of my security passes. Without them, I couldn't work.

Deeply unnerved by this uncharacteristic mental lapse, I leaned against the wall. Is this the beginning of a meltdown? I wondered. Maybe I'm just in denial about how I'm handling this loss and this work. Maybe I have to admit that it's really getting to me . . . that I just can't do it.

Pulling myself together, I called a colleague at the office, described my situation, confided in her about my personal loss, said that I'd be at least two hours late, and headed back to the Metro. After a few stops, the train halted. There had been an incident at Gallery Place. Someone had committed suicide by jumping in front of a train. Subway service was being curtailed. Besides being a terrible tragedy for the person involved, this meant that, if I wanted to get back to work, I would have to drive.

Can I trust myself to do it? I fretted over whether I could muster the needed concentration and coordination. But I made myself get into the car and go. Arriving more than two hours late, I called the remote telepsychiatry location to start the session.

"Sgt. Johnson is here," said the secretary. "His appointment was supposed to start thirty minutes ago. He's demanding to see you, even if it's only for a few minutes. He seems agitated."

I remembered Sgt. Johnson well. He had been deployed in Iraq at least twice. He'd described seeing his best buddy get killed by a handmade bomb; the memory still gave him nightmares.

After his first deployment, he'd returned to a drug-addicted father who was dying in the hospital. Deployed again, he was brought back home after his mother developed cancer. He'd spent eight months taking care of her as she wasted away; she'd died in his arms. He had recently attended a criminal trial in which one of his siblings had been convicted and sent to prison.

Johnson's psychiatric sufferings reflected his real-life traumas: anxiety, hyperalertness, sleeplessness, agitation, irritability, depression, intrusive thoughts. You name it, he had it.

Now, he was demanding to see me. I had no idea what to expect; was he angry that I was late?

Apprehensively, I sat down in front of the monitor and logged on. Sgt. Johnson appeared on the screen.

"Doc, I just want to say that the medication you gave me is really helping. My wife and I were able to go to a movie recently for the first time in years."

He looked straight at me. "Also, I want to tell you how sorry I am for the loss of your mother yesterday . . . I think you have real courage, showing up today."

How did he know? I wondered, and then realized that my colleague must have shared the news.

Conflicting emotions engulfed me: lingering embarrassment and guilt over my lateness; relief that, rather than being irate, the sergeant was eager to express his appreciation for how much better he was doing; and astonished gratitude that such a courageous man would consider me courageous.

In that moment, I couldn't convey any of this, but there was no need. He could see that I was speechless.

Finally, I managed to say, "Thank you."

And that is why I work with soldiers.

## PROFESSIONAL REFLECTIONS

There is so much to be gained by association with soldiers. For months, I had been ministering to this soldier about his reactions to death—first about watching his buddy being killed with a handmade bomb and then watching his mother die in his arms.

Now, suddenly and unexpectedly, I found myself being ministered to by him following the death of my mother. United in our mutual reactions to death, I was speechless that this hero thought of me as courageous for coming to work. His generous offer of support in my grief gave new meaning to my life.

Learning about the moral dilemmas and traumas faced by soldiers can enlarge one's moral universe. I cannot guarantee that you will have a similar experience as mine, but I can guarantee that your moral universe will expand by learning about the moral traumas faced by soldiers who are dedicating their lives to protecting us.

# PART VI

# RECRUITING: A NECESSARY TASK?

CHAPTER TWENTY-ONE

# HOW DOES ONE UNDERSTAND THE MISUNDERSTOOD?

As soon as I arrived at work, the clinical coordinator said he had some information I should know, but he was not certain he wanted to tell me.

"If I don't need to know, don't tell me."

"You have to know." Then he proceeded to tell me that one of my patients committed suicide a few days ago. I had not seen him in a year and a half, but as soon as I glanced at my notes, I remembered everything about him. Who could forget the intensity of that man's rage? He was angry with everyone.

He had a plan to kill his parents. Actually, one was a stepparent. His mother had died in his arms when he was ten years old. He could not determine how to kill his parents without being caught, so he was trying to figure out a way for someone else to do it.

He and his girlfriend had two children while living with his parents. They had objected to him selling illegal drugs out of their house and kicked him out. Then they sued for custody of his daughters and won. When I first saw this man, he had just returned from court, where he had entered into an angry confrontation with the judge. His children seemed to be the only people with whom he had a positive attachment.

I was concerned about his homicidal behavior, but I never had an indication of possible suicide. How had this situation changed? He told me that, as a single parent, he could not get into the Army. He had married his girlfriend to be eligible for enlistment. He despised her and was now trying to get rid of her as well as his parents. Furthermore, he was in administrative trouble with his commanding officer. His anger was uncontainable. Now, after his death, the only honorable thing to do was to review his chart and see what happened.

Initially, I wondered how someone "this fractured" gets into the military. Clearly, he had thought that service in the Army would help him get his life together. It is true that recruiters may extend a wide net to enlist or ensnare broken *and* unbroken youth. Belonging to the Army often helps a young person to form an identity. Over generations, nearly every family in America has a problem child—often lacking proper discipline. A time in the Army, families believe, may fill in the holes and provide the strength and stability that the family could not.

Before I started working in telepsychiatry, my knee-jerk reaction was to blame the recruiters. After all, they have quotas and allegedly make promises to enlistees they cannot fulfill. Yet, the unsuspecting recruit does not really understand what the mission of the Army actually means in the light of personal choice.

After I met some recruiters as patients, I changed my mind. As with all aspects of war, there is more complexity than at first appears. Recruiters are decent people under enormous pressure to meet quotas. Many are assigned the job with no particular training. The pressure rises for the recruiter with each passing month. I had no idea that, as a group, recruiters have one of the highest suicide rates in the military.

While recruiting, the recruiters are not deployed; obviously, nor have the men and women being recruited been deployed. Yet, one third of all suicides occur among soldiers who have never been deployed. Why do these men and women kill themselves? Clearly, it is not just the rigors of combat.

Looking back through my notes on this soldier, I see that as a young boy he was living with his mother after his parents divorced. I remember asking him what happened to him after she died of a chronic illness when he was ten. "I lived in the parks," he said. Years later, a family took him in. He lived a short time with one of his grandparents but left after he was abused. He witnessed a murder. He saw a woman get hit by a car traveling at seventy miles per hour. Most of his peers were in jail, but he got a GED and joined the Army.

This past year and a half had been problematic. He had been referred for a Medical Evaluation Board and was told he had four mental health diagnoses. Yet, my review indicated that an even bigger problem might have been his physical pain. He was taking a sleeping medication for which one of the side effects was sleepwalking. His wife tried to wake him up unsuccessfully. Unable to convince him that he was sleepwalking, she used her cell phone to make a movie of it. Recently, he had fallen down the stairs and broken some bones. The pain had registered an excruciating ten out of ten. Opioids were only modestly helpful. Many visits to pain clinics had made no significant difference.

During the time when he was seeking treatment for his fractures and physical pain, he began missing his mental health appointments. He received phone calls and letters, all while reassuring his counselor that he would keep his next appointment. When the next appointment was missed, another one was scheduled.

He had a normal physical examination by his regular physician just days before his death. "No concerns noted" was the exact observation. Then he killed himself. The emergency room record shows that they worked very hard to save him.

With his history, I wonder when he actually died or when his life ended. Was it at age ten when his mother died in his arms or later when one of his grandparents abused him? Or was it while watching the murder? Or when he was kicked out of his parents' house? Or when he lost custody of his children?

Some things are so broken even the US Army cannot repair them. Maybe his recruiter was just trying to be helpful. This soldier was not a likeable person, but where would he have learned how to be liked?

## PROFESSIONAL REFLECTIONS

The Army needs to replenish its soldiers each year. Since the elimination of the selective service, serving in the military has become the home of a more specifically selected group of people. Joining the military is an alternative for high school graduates who choose it or delay going to college. Many individuals, while serving in the military, pursue education in college and beyond.

Traditionally, adolescents who need structure and discipline or who are indecisive about their future have joined the military as a rite of passage or just a maturing experience. The military has become much more than the above as it currently offers multiple career paths, educational and health benefits, and a way "to see the world." "Be all that you can be" is an attractive marketing slogan.

There are multiple examples of the military "turning a life around." We expect a great deal from our military. Repairing every broken civilian life is more than it can do.

# CHAPTER TWENTY-TWO

# RESPONDING TO THE CALL

Haven't you always wondered why young men and women join the military? After all, they do have a choice. Most of us who are older did not, unless going to jail or going to Canada were your other options.

It is not always strictly part of the medical history, but I do ask that question of the soldiers, sailors, Marines, pilots, privates, and field grade officers I see. When did you join? How far out of high school were you? What were your reasons? Did you go to college? If so, did you take ROTC? What did you think you would accomplish?

The answers have some similarities, some differences, and many are quite remarkable. Some decisions are impulsive. Many responses reflect a plan or strategy for a new life. Some are based on multigenerational family traditions. There are individuals who know from an early age that they want to serve their country as a soldier. Some of them are like the young people who know they want to be first responders. They want to serve others and be in dangerous, challenging situations. They take every opportunity to prove themselves physically fit and fit to handle challenges. Many had fathers and grandfathers who did the same thing. Often, one of their ancestors was among the fallen. They see themselves as continuing the family tradition. It is remarkable to watch and, unfortunately for our protection, society needs these people.

Sometimes, the people in charge of those sent out to protect us come to see me. They know—and often on a daily basis—that a certain number of the men and women they deploy will not return. Each night, a patrol leaves with some who will not be coming back. Sometimes, the cause is enemy fire, and sometimes, it has been a "friendly" mistake. Always being aware, however, does not keep these leaders from sending the soldiers. It is a certain type of leader who can decrease awareness in order to keep deploying soldiers. Some speak of the "pain" of knowing that each night one of the few they select will not return. Others prefer just to live and act and not speak of what lies deep in their minds.

There are soldiers who are exposed to dangerous fire from the first moment of deployment. Every day, every night, and all day long, they must watch and be aware. They take turns and depend on one another. When working with indigenous personnel, it is often difficult to distinguish the indigenous from the insurgents. So, they must learn to watch even those who are helping them. What happens to a brain and mind that constantly focuses on danger twenty-four hours a day, 365 days a year? As you can well imagine, that brain eventually forgets how to turn itself off. After a year's exposure to constantly anticipating danger, the brain responds to anything that startles, even from a newborn child. Middle of the night noises or cries can arouse a soldier to gather his or her civilian family into the basement preparing for an attack. To be fair, this reaction is extreme but not rare.

As I listen to soldiers, I have become more aware of the different responses between direct and indirect combat. When you can look the enemy in the eye, you know with whom you are dealing. It may be a kill or be killed situation. The adrenaline flows, but there is certain clarity in the task at hand. Some soldiers describe it as exhilarating. The calmness of civilian life cannot compare.

Indirect fire is much more arbitrary. Rockets, mortars, IEDs.

When will they come, how often, who will be hit? Anyone and everyone at any time can be hit. Will I be a target or will the person next to me or will we all survive? "The randomness is worse than the direct confrontation," says one soldier. "The impact washes over you. When will the next one come?" Arbitrariness and uncertainty for most of us is much more difficult than the known. Our brains, the biological substrate of our minds, become sensitized to this episodic alternating of certainty and uncertainty. When will it come? Here it is. Will it be me? Sometimes, it is better to not have time to think.

Soldiers bring their reactions home. Their reactions are not left on the battlefield. Often, the ones with no physical injury and just the mental injury get the least sympathy. I have heard many stories, but sometimes one just stands out.

Recently, a soldier referred for medication told me of his deployment experiences and the related nightmares and anxiety attacks. Courageously, he preferred to deal with these reactions with methods of self-regulation and not medication. He practiced meditation and performed biofeedback exercises and mindfulness exercises. He and his wife began looking for a new church for worship. She preferred a more avant-garde form of worship. He was looking for a more reserved form. He yielded, and one Sunday they went to a church with a band.

The church was a large room, rather crowded, and so "it felt like a confined space." The band was loud with a particularly vibrant bass violin. As they began, the music filled the room and he could experience vibrations in the air, then in his chest, and then in his mind. Each time the bass struck a vibrant chord, he would get a quick visual image. The louder the music, the stronger the shockwaves in the air, and the more intense the image. One moment, he was in the church and the next in the battle and then the church and then the battle. It was as if there were arbitrary explosions going off all over the room. Each chord brought another vibration, another explosion, and another image. He had to leave.

After these experiences, he said he was not himself for a period of time. "How so?" I asked. "Did you ever get into an argument with your wife over toilet paper at Walmart?" he said. I got his point. His brain got so aroused and irritated that his mind was agitated about things that make no difference. Paradoxically, his brain was so reactive to one stimulus that his mind was unable to function in other areas. It became hard to be reasonable even about toilet paper. To his credit and that of his family's, he was able to spend some time, as he frequently does, in self-regulation and rejoin the family later in the day. We have all heard of the soldiers who cannot participate in July Fourth activities because of the explosions. How many of us know soldiers that find it hard to worship in a church because of their combat experiences?

## PROFESSIONAL REFLECTIONS

This soldier, or one like him, may be a member of your religious congregation, your place of employment, or even a neighbor. Treating him just as a hero is a disservice to his experience and his service. He is having trouble being a "normal" spouse. Many like him are having trouble being "normal" fathers. His world feels as if it is not safe. His moral, spiritual, and physical recovery depends on finding a safe and predictable community.

If you see him or her, find a way to make them feel welcomed. Studies suggest that even random acts of kindness are helpful. Providing a "normal" civilian experience can be an important step to recovery.

Previous societies, in particular the Greeks, had community rituals after wars for returning soldiers and civilians. Greek tragic plays were performed so that soldiers and civilians could share a common sense of tragedy. The assumption that "we are all in this together" seems to have been lost in our society. Unless our civilians help soldiers manage their trauma, soldiers who fought in our stead will carry all the grief and anguish for our country—the ultimate moral betrayal.

## CHAPTER TWENTY-THREE

# HER PROBLEM SHOULD BE OURS

My job is to help soldiers do their jobs. A large part of that work entails making them deployable—ready for war. Although not a pleasant metaphor, they are like missiles—instruments of war, ready for war. Yet, unlike missiles, soldiers are reusable. My job is treating the effects of their war experiences so that the soldiers can be reused. When they are suffering or are impaired by war, the goal is to improve their functioning so that they can be redeployed. If not deployable, they may be medically discharged from the service. I am well aware of how war affects them. I am *growing* in awareness of how our civilian society impedes the functioning of soldiers.

Soldiers are on the front line in military conflicts. Much has been written about these experiences. Yet, we have known for a long time that 99 percent of society knows little about the 1 percent who carry on our wars. Recently, I was surprised to learn that soldiers can be on the front line in societal civilian issues as well. These problems are ones created by civilians who can influence and affect the military; while not necessarily violent, they may become so. These stories are not so widely known. Civilian conflicts, unlike military conflicts, are not necessarily violent but may become so.

These civilian societal problems are often an outgrowth of the way society organizes and confronts evolving social issues. These issues may involve guns, violence, and discrepancies in income and education. Immigration policy, as well as a bellicose foreign policy, may not be sufficiently supported by money and manpower. How do soldiers, employed by the military, become negatively affected when they come in contact with civilian policies? Let's look at the work of one recruiter whom I recently interviewed.

The interview instantly brought me face to face with these issues. This soldier recently purchased her own gun for protection. I asked why she felt it necessary and from whom she was seeking protection. "A fellow soldier," she replied. A few years ago, as a commander of a unit at another base, she had disciplined this soldier. He blamed her for his subsequent problems. He posted threats to kill her on social media. He was hospitalized, treated, and discharged. He apparently remained threatening. Even though my patient had been transferred to another base, she remained traumatized by this experience. The threatening soldier was separated from the military but lived in a state that allowed his purchase of guns. Hence, my patient felt it necessary to buy a weapon for protection against the former soldier. Living with this potential threat, the trauma was reinforced by having a gun in her own home. Soldiers, trained to be killers, sometimes adapt poorly to civilian life. A change in our gun policies might make this stalker less threatening. My patient is clearly threatened by the availability of guns to her stalker and to herself.

The patient continues her job as a recruiter. "It is a 'numbers' game," she says. She has to get a certain number of persons to commit to the service each month. If she does not meet her quota, she can be penalized. The pressure is intense. She is anxious and depressed. She also knows that recruiters have a high rate of suicide.

To do her job, this recruiter offers high school students an educational future, potential job security, travel benefits, free medical care, potential retirement benefits, and an opportunity "to be all that you can be." She travels to high schools in wealthy suburban communities to recruit qualified students. Parents are allowed to "check a box" to prevent their sons and daughters from having contact with recruiters. In these upper and middle class neighborhoods, the parents readily "check the box." They want their kids to have no access to recruiters. She waits in the office and no one comes, no one signs up. These students have an educational future, potential job security, free travel, as well as medical and potential retirement benefits. However, these parents have decided that no wartime service is necessary for their children. They will provide. But when these parents provide, rather than expose their children to national service, have they deprived them of something important?

So, my patient is forced to go to high schools in geographical areas where the "future is not so certain." Negating to check the box, these parents readily check "yes" for recruiter access to their children. Immigrants are willing to serve even if they are not citizens. Our "volunteer" Army is recruited from these disadvantaged areas of society. Sometimes, these students are not qualified. They may not pass the physical and mental tests. What does a recruiter do?! We have had a war in Iraq and Afghanistan, and some of us want one in Syria. So, we need soldiers. Often, those less qualified students, relatively speaking, are willing to volunteer as they are looking for a "leg up" in society.

The rules get changed. Students with poor grades, or students who are obese and out of shape or who have used drugs or who have criminal records, are selected and sent to basic training. Some have felt that the front line was a lot safer than living in their high school neighborhoods. Some of these recruits make it through basic and advanced training and some do not. Some have a career "as promised."

My patient, the recruiter, gets her monthly numbers from this population for the most part. She remains, however, quite anxious and unsatisfied. She worries about "the numbers" game. She was brought up in a leadership culture that cared about a soldier's personal and family life. She works nightly and most weekends. There is no time for herself and her family or "fun stuff." She is a little puzzled as to how difficult society has made her recruiting job for wars that the same society says it wants.

I think I understand society's ambivalence. But when does an ambivalent society become an irresponsible society? I know I was very ambivalent about serving when drafted into the Army in 1967. Ultimately, I felt I could not be a conscientious objector because I reached that position only when faced with the draft. Now, we all check that recruiting box that says, "No contact with my children." Our middle class young adults are not only being kept from speaking with soldiers who serve but shielded from the entire concept of national service to our country as a whole.

Yes, I know many serve in soup kitchens, but there are wars going on, threats of terrorist attacks, and tens of thousands of displaced refugees. Yet, we are unwittingly standing in the way of the soldiers whom we have asked to protect us. Talking to this recruiter made the issue loud and clear. What do we as a community—parents, teachers, school boards, and educators—think and want to do?

Service, if not as a citizen soldier, then at least as a citizen of national service, should be mandatory. We owe it to ourselves, our children, and to this recruiter.

## PROFESSIONAL REFLECTIONS

**National service might facilitate the reduction of our current "tribalism" and our estrangement from one another. It accomplishes this by expanding familiarity of youth with persons not part of their families, schools, or immediate neighborhood, and instead national service offers youths the opportunity to be depended upon rather than to be dependent. The case for *National Service: What Would It Mean?* has been made by Richard**

Danzig and Peter Szanton. Senators, former Secretary of Defense Robert McNamara, and various college presidents have endorsed their book and research published in 1986. They propose various types of national service, voluntary and universal, designed to meet unmet social and personal needs. Only one of their various plans involves military service.

The authors provide arguments about why national service may or may not work. One persistent attraction of national service is providing youths a broader experience in life. Service that required sacrifice, intensive effort, and some risk might offer a sense of citizenship earned—in other words, one had paid one's dues. The authors argue that currently only veterans, Peace Corps volunteers, and immigrant citizens have a sense of citizenship earned. Since the publication of their work, small pilot programs in our nation's high schools have sprung up, requiring service learning for graduation to be successful.

National service has the potential for citizens to relearn the importance of service for the common good. Citizen understanding and familiarity of the service of our military men and women would be a solid step in that direction.

# CHAPTER TWENTY-FOUR

# RECRUITING REVISITED

Until I started working regularly with servicemen and women, I never focused much on my negative bias against military recruiters. How could anyone try to talk young kids into voluntarily putting themselves in harm's way! What kind of people would do this? I have learned that it is a more complex issue.

In the past, the concept of service was not controversial. Like many people, I grew up expecting that everyone would volunteer for service to our country. Some of us went into the Peace Corps, others volunteered in domestic programs, and many of us went into the military. I remember getting that letter in August 1967 from President Lyndon B. Johnson telling me I would arrive at Tan Son Nhut Air Base in Saigon wearing combat boots and khakis. There was no discussion and no enticement.

The political implementation of the draft, however, was controversial. One joined the military as a part of being a citizen of the country, but the system failed to enforce the draft equitably. One could avoid it by getting married, having children, going to college, knowing the right people, or having a political connection. I even explored being a conscientious objector, but I reasoned that entering as a physician meant I was supporting soldiers and not the direct war effort.

Service to the country has been replaced by other considerations. Young men and women like the challenge presented by the military. The money, a job with a benefits package, and college tuition are added incentives. Patriotism is a distant third. These changes make recruitment more difficult. How did we get here?

Richard Nixon ran for president during the middle of the war. When he was advised that his support of the draft was unpopular, he switched to supporting an all-volunteer Army.

The result: To fight subsequent wars, and now the longest war in the history of the United States, we need bodies to fight for us. Soldiers are one of our fighting instruments. They have to be managed and maintained like tanks, artillery, and missiles. If used too much, they wear out and/or get used up, and so they have to be replaced.

We need men and women specifically assigned to get young people to sign contracts for service in dangerous places. These people are called recruiters. Young people are told about all the places they will go and things they will get "consistent with the needs of the Army." The physical challenge and the benefits package are major considerations. How can a young person understand that "consistent with the needs of the Army" really means subsuming your needs to a larger group?

Young people do routinely subsume their individuality when they marry for a lifetime. Is subsuming your individuality to the military any different? Few people really understand what they are getting into in either situation. Subsuming "for love" rather than subsuming "for war" seems more comprehensible if not more romantic.

The military needs recruits to continue its mission. If, as our society believes it is necessary to have a standing and engaged military around the world, then it needs people willing to fight. As long as our society believes fighting with others is better than cooperating with others, our society will need people to fight. We should not kid ourselves, because these recruiters work for us—we, the 99 percent who do not have to be involved directly in the war efforts. I have learned that many recruiters do not like that idea any more than we do.

Service as a recruiter can be compulsory. It can be a condition for future promotion. Some branches of the service require the top percentage of soldiers in a group to compete for a position as a recruiter that none of them want. They are "*voluntold* rather than volunteered."

In some ways, this recruiting service is antithetical to their basic training. In basic training, they are taught survival as a cohesive, centralized altruistic group. As recruiters, they are required to be a cohesive but decentralized group that competes against one another. They are spread out over a geographic area, working on their own to fill assigned quotas. It is like a "bad statistics class." They have to make a fixed number of phone calls to generate a certain number of appointments with a percentage yield that garners one recruit. Day after day, month after month, they have to produce. Their cars have reverse GPSs, and phone calls are monitored. The military keeps track of what they are doing. Lacking the familiar hierarchical military structure, however, recruiters are on their own and often get into trouble. Pressure to produce promotes misconduct. Recently, *The Washington Post* reported that a local Maryland recruiter developed an intimate relationship with a female high school recruit. This problem resulted in a homicide and suicide. He killed her and himself.

While recruiting, they are able to avoid the stress of deployment. Yet, in some branches of the service they have one of the highest suicide rates in the military. Recruiters have to explain why it is desirable to be one of these instruments of war, the value of being part of a group that will eventually become more concerned about you than you are about yourself. This learned altruism is an enticing experience for young people or for anyone at any age. It may be particularly attractive to this younger generation that we older ones often think are more self-centered than we are.

The dilemmas remain; the complexity is there. The job is difficult. I am more sympathetic to recruiters now that I know some. Recently, one told me that he stood on a high school graduation stage and offered an $80,000 scholarship package for recruits that included college benefits and more. An enticing proposal! The two speakers who followed the recruiter were a mother and father whose daughter served in Afghanistan. They offered a $1,000 college scholarship in her memory.

Which scholarship would you want?

Recruiting: Not an easy job!

## PROFESSIONAL REFLECTIONS

This recruiter is struggling with our societal residue of the Vietnam War. The war was unwinnable in part because its goal was unclear. Charting victory by a public policy of counting dead bodies was incompatible with "winning the hearts and minds" of the people. Our government concealed these facts from the American public, which led to countrywide protests. Many middle- and upper-class kids in college obtained deferments. Many lower socioeconomic, non-married non-students went to war. Returning soldiers were poorly treated by society, especially those opposed to the war. Parents whose children went to war were more supportive. As a cultural divide, the societal residue of the Vietnam War ensued and persists today.

Richard Nixon determined that the elimination of the selective service draft meant that your sons would no longer have to die in Vietnam. It was determined that Nixon's action would decrease the protest.

The recruiter described in this essay struggles with both issues: 1) the cultural divide and 2) the all-voluntary Army. Almost no one protests the continuation of our unending war. Almost everyone is satisfied with someone else's children fighting these wars. Serving in the military is an honorable profession, but it can be dangerous. If 99 percent of our population does not want to participate in the military in order to protect our common good, they at least have an obligation to know more about our soldiers and to serve the common good in some other manner.

These volunteer soldiers are joining the military in part to protect us, our moral and physical space, to allow civilians to work together on the common good as we see fit. When they return and want to rejoin our space, we as citizens are obligated to welcome and to listen to any moral harm soldiers have incurred while defending us. To the extent that they can tell their stories, we must find a way to listen.

CHAPTER TWENTY-FIVE

# A RETIRING RECRUITER LOOKS BACK

Soldiers retire, some after long careers. Helping them with their transition plans allows them to review their careers as well as the changing nature of the Army. I have been treating a soldier in charge of a specialized warfare program who recently made the decision to retire. His physical condition made participation in the current planned field exercises too difficult. It was not easy for him to decide voluntarily. He knew, however, that not participating was in his long-term health's best interests. His unit would miss him, and he clearly knew his own misgivings. To plan for his absence, he developed a manual with diagrams, instructions, and photos with which he believed everyone would know what to do in his absence. Standing or sitting in a room, this soldier radiates competence.

There's no doubt about his confidence and certainty, despite an edge of disquiet that he partially revealed in his first appointment. Initially, he was very concerned about the genetically based disease of one of his children. The child was adjusting very well. But he clearly "felt guilty" about "causing" the child's problem. His feelings were profound and irrational. Trying to explore the nature of his guilt, I asked about his command experience. "How many soldiers have you lost in battle?"

"A number of them," he said.

"Do you feel responsible?" I asked.

"Not at all. It is just part of the job," he replied.

Watching him, I puzzled over figuring out how to put those two responses together. Then even more puzzling, I saw tears on his face.

We had talked several times about his guilt, and I was never certain "where he was." Now, in our last session, I asked, "Where are you going to retire?"

"I am moving back to the republic," he said. "God, country, family, and where I can carry a gun all the time. And I'm not afraid to use it," he added. Somehow, I knew he was talking about Texas. I spent two years in the military in San Antonio and learned that Texans could not understand why anyone would ever want to leave their state.

Soon, he spoke of something else niggling at his brain. His physical problems were not the only reason for his retirement. Rather, the direction "the Army was moving" was also a factor. He worried about the Army's policies on recruitment. He had been a recruiter for years, knew the problems in recruiting, and even acknowledged that he, like his colleagues, had "cut corners." He said it's a matter of numbers. Every recruiter had to produce new people. "When the deadline arrives and the quota is unmet, even convicted felons are recruited." He admitted to bringing in unqualified candidates to make his quota. He believed that if he did not take some of the "unqualified," another recruiter would take them. Besides, he wanted to go home and be with his wife at seven p.m. rather than ten p.m. each night.

Recently, he became upset about the Army's decision to admit transgender recruits. He denied any personal prejudice but stated that sooner or later they will make a decision about surgery and, during an extensive recovery period, they would not be eligible for deployment. Since readiness for deployment is "key" in the Army, he could not understand why the Army would admit people whom they knew would not be deployable. Apparently, he assumed that all transgender soldiers would have surgery and that the recovery and rehabilitation period was extensive. The military was planning to require transgender recruits to have been stable in their new genders for eighteen months.

Knowing the Army had just instituted a mandatory transgender sensitization course for "everyone," I asked what he was doing about that. He said that he explained his position and refused to take the course. "Are you in any trouble?" I asked.

"Not so far," he replied. He complained further about the sense of entitlement and lack of resilience in the current generation. One purpose of basic training, he often stated, was to identify personal weaknesses and then correct them. He acknowledged he was "old school" and that every generation probably has doubts about the next generation. "Some recruits now completing basic training found it so difficult that they were claiming PTSD," he said. He acknowledged that routine basic training might cause trainees to complain to their parents, who then complain to their congressman, who complains to the generals, who make it known to the drill instructors. So, he believes, individuals who fail basic training are just continually recycled to another training unit until the Army finds one they can pass.

I have no way to vouch for or verify his claims about basic training, but his story about being a drill instructor fascinated me. He recounted that one day marching back to camp and calling out the usual cadence, his troops were not very responsive. The commander of the unit said, "This will not do. It must be changed and by tomorrow." At that directive, my drill sergeant patient told the commander to leave the area so the latter would have plausible deniability. He then marched the troops over to the sand pit. "One learns in the Army by repetition or blunt force," the drill sergeant said. He explained that over the next four hours, he demanded that the troops perform continuous, intense, and unrelenting exercises. "I never touched anyone," he added. "The trainees were so exhausted, we had to carry some back to camp. But there were no further problems."

Personally, I am opposed to war. I believe the world will progress more effectively through cooperation rather than conflict. I cannot imagine going through "real" basic training. I do not know if I were in a "kill or be killed" situation if I could kill another person. I am too aware of the "consequences of living" after having inflicted trauma on another human being. I thought, and almost said aloud, if I were in combat and in a foxhole, I would want this soldier and the troops he trained to be with me. He said, "God bless you" when we said goodbye. A complicated individual, this recruiter is both sincere and impenetrable.

## PROFESSIONAL REFLECTIONS

This soldier has a lot to teach us. His competence is contagious. He has strong, clear opinions. He worked cooperatively for years with others with whom he differed. He has problems with the current changes in the military, in particular the service of transgender individuals. While undergoing surgery, he believes, transgender individuals would not be deployable for a mission. His objections to their service are more medical than personal. His service continued.

The Army also has a lot to teach us. They are recommending the continuing service of transgender individuals. A Rand Corporation study states there are about "1,320 and 6,630 transgender service members among 1.3 million on active duty, less than 1 per cent of the force." The Army convinces many different types of people to "Be all you can be."

In conjunction with the above study, Marine Gen. Joseph F. Dunford Jr., chairman of the Joint Chiefs of Staff, directed "that all people will be 'treated with dignity and respect.'" In keeping with that tradition, the American military is the "most racially integrated institution in the world." According to Leonard Steinhorn of American University, our military has the highest rate of racial intermarriage and our military bases have the most racially integrated neighborhoods in America.

I am pleased that individuals like this soldier are dedicated to making us safer. There is a lot for civilians to learn from the military about how to live together in service of the common good.

[illegible] and investigations and our military bases have, the [illegible] [illegible] concluded.

[illegible] nothing is [illegible]

# PART VII

# LEADERSHIP

# CHAPTER TWENTY-SIX
# GETTING THINGS DONE?

Most of my time with soldiers is problem focused. Psychiatrists and physicians are trained to identify and help solve problems. Occasionally, I get to just sit back and watch interesting events unfold. Such was the situation recently with a very responsible field grade officer.

Janet did not occupy the leadership position she desired. Her initial complaints centered on not being promoted. She was working with people who "endlessly recycled unworkable solutions." Her frustration and irritation were high. I suspected her of being an *overfunctioner*, a person who does her share of work and the work of others. Clearly, she was a "take charge" person who was frustrated by being unable to do so in her current assignment.

Is Janet's leadership typical of Army leadership? I do not know. I do know that the Army is a hierarchical organization where leaders issue commands and soldiers unquestionably follow them for the good of the group. One's life depends on one's brother or sister, and his or her life depends on the other. It is a reciprocal agreement to protect another with your life; it is not negotiable. The loss of another is more drastic than the prospect of one's own death.

Janet seemed pleased to vent her job frustration, and I was sympathetic to the dilemmas presented. Is there a difference between being responsible *to* others rather than being responsible *for* others? Then came the big problem. Her sister who lived a thousand miles away was pregnant, unmarried, beyond the "safe age" for childbearing, and hospitalized in a mental hospital.

Their father with whom her sister lived had just died. Janet's sister was in a behavioral regression and hearing voices.

Janet was distressed and uncertain about how to proceed. Her leadership focus was always on taking responsibility no matter the circumstances. Contact with her sister was not initially productive. Janet contacted the father of the child, a local handyman who wanted no part of the pregnancy. Efforts to communicate with her sister's mental health team ran up against HIPAA, those annoying federal guidelines that prevent even common sense communication between family and patient caregivers.

Janet traveled to visit her sister and settle their father's estate, as well as sell the house where they both had lived. Her sister did not want an abortion but had limited ability to care for a child if and when she was discharged from the hospital. As the pregnancy progressed, she was discharged and planned to place the child up for adoption.

Janet discussed these developments for weeks and months. She became progressively convinced that she did not want to see her prospective niece or nephew (family) "lost" to the foster care or adoption system. She discussed her concerns with her sister with little resolution.

Eventually, Janet's sister gave birth to a daughter, my patient's niece. The mother left the obstetrics hospital, but the child did not. The staff did not believe the mother could properly care for the child. Months went by while social service and child protection teams debated the proper course of action. Social services filed a petition to take the child away from the mother. Progressively upset by these actions or inactions, my patient joined the court proceedings and filed for temporary custody of the child. The judge, preferring that the girl stay within the family, granted her petition. Knowing my patient worked full time, I continued to ask if her spouse fully supported her action, and she assured me he did.

Janet was determined not to "lose" her niece in the foster care or adoption system. Her spouse agreed to help, and they implemented a plan. Personally, I did not think it was the best idea—to take a child from her hospitalized sister and bring her home to their house. My patient worked full time and had adult children. Months went by, and Janet realized that the niece was beginning to become quite attached to her while the baby's birth mother remained hundreds of miles away in and out of the hospital "getting mental health treatment."

My patient accomplished her goal but eventually decided the "victory" was a mixed blessing. She had assumed all the responsibility for the care of this child while her sister remained in treatment. The uncertainty of whether her sister would ever assume care for her child was disturbing to Janet, who was used to everything being in its proper place. Janet wondered if hearing voices created problems with being a parent. "Not necessarily," I commented while noting that a number of people with schizophrenia were good parents.

Frustrated with her inability to communicate with her sister's treatment team and get a timeline for reuniting mother and child, Janet made a bold proposal. She and her spouse would drive to this distant city, pick up her sister, and move her to Janet's home. There, her sister would be offered a place to stay, assistance in raising her daughter, and treatment by a local county mental health team. Janet put the pieces in place and discussed it with her sister, who agreed to come.

Janet announced that she would pick up her sister at noon on a specific day. She expected her to be packed and ready and asked for help from "friends who owed Janet favors." She called and told them to get her sister ready "by the expected time." Halfway through the trip, Janet called and said she was on the way. At eleven a.m. on the appointed day, Janet left a message saying she would be there at noon. Fifty-eight minutes later, at two minutes to twelve, she texted, "I am outside your house." Janet told her sister that if she did not come with her and take responsibility for raising her daughter with assistance, their relationship was over.

Her sister now lives with Janet's family. They talk at least one hour each day. Janet tells her sister's voices to behave themselves. If they do not she "will kick them out of the house." Asking me what I thought, I told her that it was a rather unique approach. I advised that when she met with her sister's mental health team that she "be cautious" before confiding all that she was doing. Her leadership, this take charge posture, seemed a little unorthodox for the situation.

Months went by with almost every piece in place. Janet ponders the one piece that she cannot control: that her sister "does not seem to know how to be a mom."

MISSION ACCOMPLISHED? We will see! There may be limits to what one can expect "military leadership" to accomplish—not only in war, but in peace, foreign policy, and personal relationships.

## PROFESSIONAL REFLECTIONS

**Janet's situation provided an opportunity to observe the application of a military field grade officer's skills to a "family" problem. Janet appeared to be a take-charge-over-functioning type of leader. Not being recently promoted may have been related to her leadership style, but she had achieved significant status as a lieutenant colonel.**

**For the Army, the loss of another is more drastic than the prospect of one's own death. Janet saw the loss of her niece to another family as equally drastic. Our military has impressive leadership skills for short-term interventions. Janet demonstrated those skills as she improvised a rather unorthodox manner of getting her niece transferred out of the hospital, away from her allegedly incompetent mother and away from child protective services and into Janet's home.**

Janet accomplished her goal but eventually decided the "victory" was a mixed blessing. Her niece's mother, Janet's sister, was still in the hospital a thousand miles away. Janet devised a successful stealth operation that brought her sister into her home to care for the child.

Months went by with almost every piece in place. Janet pondered, after "victory," the one piece that she could not control: that her sister "does not seem to know how to be a mom."

Janet's family leadership matter has parallels with military leadership regarding our invasion of Iraq. Our American military is designed for short, decisive campaigns and not for protracted counterinsurgencies designed to win the hearts and minds of the people. The military leaders define the problem, get a "green light" from the administration, and take over and solve it. Once our victory in Iraq was declared, Iraq still did not know how to govern itself. Janet, applying her military skills, saved her sister's child, but her sister had no idea about the long haul and how to be the child's mother. There may be limits to what one can expect "military leadership" to accomplish!

Our American public should be asking questions of our public officials and military leaders. What is the purpose of solving an alleged problem, and should we be doing so, just because our political leaders think they know how to do it? As former Marine and bestselling author Phil Klay suggests, we should not be collecting scalps just because we can do so.

Klay further opines, "If I have authority to speak about our military policy it's because I'm a citizen responsible for participating in self-government, not because I belonged to a warrior caste." A first step for each citizen in knowing more about these issues might be getting to know more soldiers, their experience and their mission. It is an important step citizens can take in exercising their obligation to support the common good and to acknowledge we are all working on this country together.

# CHAPTER TWENTY-SEVEN
# FOLLOW THE LEADER?

Leadership is easier to think about than to execute. Everyone has an opinion about what leaders should do, and the choices are myriad. The Army has its way based on loyalty and taking care of one's buddy, a very hierarchical form of altruism. When I first began working with soldiers at the Walter Reed, I was pretty impressed with the "trappings." The flag, the uniforms, saluting one another, the discipline, the ceremonies, and rituals all contribute to the *esprit de corps* and following the leader. Watching so many amputees negotiate the cafeteria on their own is truly inspiring.

I suspect my reaction was similar to that of the many young people who join the military. The singular focus of leaders, the patriotism, "fighting our enemies," the glory and valor, and the strangely comforting identification with all of it can obscure vision. In retrospect, I think the inspiration I experienced led to my overlooking some obvious problems in the military leadership of our unit. I believe a similar process overtakes young soldiers. They may not really understand what they are getting into. I don't think I did either, but there is a difference. I could walk away from my problematic leader, but they cannot. Their job is to follow a command without questioning.

Although their mission is organized around altruism, ironically, their leaders do not always consider the needs of individuals. Soldiers discover that they cannot take vacations when they want, nor can they always attend the funerals of family members or even of their parents. The needs of the military prevail. Effective and understanding leaders are so critical to the functioning of a unit, but such leaders are not always available.

In the beginning, a rather charismatic former military leader led our group at Walter Reed and conveyed an ability to get things done. Our funds allegedly came directly from Congress, secure for years, and did not have to pass through the normal bureaucratic "checks and balances." Our military leader's discussions were always "visionary" but not necessarily logical and often a little contradictory. We mental health professionals talked among ourselves about how nice it sounded, but how discomforting it seemed.

Soldiers do not have the luxury of questioning. They are not allowed to talk about the leader or question the directions. If they receive contradictory commands, as they often do, they literally do not know what to do. One young woman I saw came in with panic attacks. Her history involved not being issued proper equipment. Later, she was ordered to operate her vehicle. She knew that not wearing proper equipment while operating a vehicle was a violation. But she was just obeying orders. Another part of the command filed a disciplinary action against her for operating her vehicle without proper equipment. She tried to explain, but one does not "talk back to command." Facing disciplinary proceedings in "this catch-22" situation gave her anxiety attacks.

We physicians could easily talk among ourselves about when our leader (military or not) was not making sense. The soldier with panic attacks could not do the same. She required medication to deal with her leaders. Most readers are aware of the recent shooting at Fort Hood, when Ivan Lopez shot himself and nineteen others. There was an extensive investigation. Leaders genuinely want to know why these episodes happen. I wonder how much note will be made of the fact that his leaders did not allow him to attend his mother's funeral. Undoubtedly, he "had feelings about not being able to attend." Leaders influence how individuals express their feelings. Some people get anxious, some get violent. Most everyone needs to talk it out.

Leaders also influence the effectiveness of the followers. Our mission was to provide behavioral health services over a secure Internet. Our leader's charisma could build a service—we grew from five to seventy-five people in a short time. Keeping the service logical, organized, and well maintained, however, was not part of his vision.

In our organization, there always seemed to be a technology crisis. Our unlimited funding apparently allowed him "to throw money at problems." For every type of technology failure, there seemed to be a member of the bureaucracy hired to assist. There was an information technology person for computers, several who worked on electronic medical records, another who did passwords, another on scheduling, and there was always an 800-number to call for more "advanced" problems. There were also employees who were in charge of contracts, research, property, and equipment. There was money to pay all these people.

Service members do not have the same benefits. Agree with it or not, our society has asked them to fight our wars. Their mission is to kill the enemy. They do not always have proper equipment, adequate supplies, or sufficient protection. Their military leaders cannot throw money at the problems. Their funding is limited by political leaders. In fact, when our soldiers return with "problems," there is insufficient money "thrown their way" to treat them medically, provide for their disability, and to reeducate them. Maybe our society needs a little more imagination regarding what is happening to our soldiers and how to be helpful.

Service members are always talking about waiting for orders: for reassignment, temporary training, disbanding a unit, or even discharge. The worst seems to be waiting for a disciplinary action.

They become tense, anxious, and bored with the waiting. The leader's reassignment inefficiency seems a waste of time and personnel.

Recently, our unit had a similar reassignment experience. The "old" Walter Reed where we worked was closing and moving to a new location. The original plans allowed for our initial five-member staff to have offices in the new location. The rumor was that our charismatic leader, with his own special stream of funding from Congress, had not alerted the planners of our growth. We were twelve times as big as when we started, and there was no room.

We could not go just anywhere. It had to be a secure Defense Department-authorized location with a maze of electronic and physical protection. Finally, the day arrived, and Walter Reed moved. We did not. We wondered if we would have an office that was open or closed. Where would it be? Mostly, we wondered, is this the way soldiers were treated? Did they often wait for deployment to one place, but then the battle plan changed and so they were sent elsewhere? We were tense and anxious.

Later, as the fiscal year closed, our contracts were also ending. Our leader assured us that all the appropriate planning and preparation was in place. We should expect a seamless transition to a new contract. Despite full schedules of patients, no contract appeared. Days then weeks passed. Younger professionals who were supporting families needed work and took other jobs. Those of us with other jobs just waited. My fellow psychiatrists talked about whether the "real" Army operated this way. What would it be like in a foxhole with chaos around you, not knowing if you could depend on others? We were not in danger, but we certainly operated within chaos.

Finally, we returned to work. The explanations for what transpired were too numerous to count. Who really knows what the leader either did or did not do? And then one day our visionary leader and his assistants disappeared, escorted out of their offices by uniformed service members. Then uniformed military people occupied offices throughout our building. We were about to experience the type of hierarchical structured leadership that service members experience. Had our leader experienced a better leader himself, this might not have happened.

I like working with soldiers. Their stories are fascinating and inspiring, and I know I can be helpful. But I also know that, unlike them, I can and they cannot, walk away from the "chaos" that seems to surround their work. Even more, I can think about and question the leadership and talk about it with my colleagues. I think it makes me a better follower. But, does questioning leadership like civilians can do make a soldier more effective?

## PROFESSIONAL REFLECTIONS

Civilians in the United States can participate with and debate the integrity of our political leadership just as my colleagues debated our administrative leadership. This fact makes us more morally responsible for decisions made by leadership. Soldiers are more automatically bound to obey commands of leadership and not question them. Retired Medal of Honor winner Col. Jack Jacobs says, "Soldiers may think a combat mission is stupid but their duty is to execute it." Soldiers do their job because they have to do it and to support those around them who are doing it.

Our professional group experienced interesting, rewarding, but at times distressing contradictory leadership directives. Soldiers experience similar leadership issues but with more severe consequences. Inconsistent or contradictory military commands and directives to soldiers can lead to confusing and anxiety-ridden behaviors in followers. Civilians in our democracy can discuss and refuse to obey directives. Soldiers must trust that leadership is honorable and informed. Command directives are, for the most part, nondiscussable.

Soldiers do count on citizens for debating and making informed decisions about undertaking just and moral wars. Phil Klay, author of *Redeployment*, says that soldiers rely on citizens to define a military mission that is "moral and achievable. The clarity of purpose so central to bonding men in combat cannot emerge purely from the military itself." Once war begins, soldiers just follow the leader and his or her commands. Soldiers obey commands or suffer the consequences—shame in not supporting fellow soldiers, punishment for refusal to obey, and shunning for cowardly behavior in the national defense against enemies.

When citizens say, "Thank you for your service," it suggests that we are all in this effort together and that soldiers are in fact fighting a war on our behalf. Although most citizens are not directly involved with the war, they all pay taxes and support industries that are directly involved. Democracies can debate war, but final leadership decisions are binding on all citizens. War is a collective societal responsibility.

As citizens, we have a responsibility to be informed participants with leadership but also followers with government decisions. Soldiers are most effective in unquestioningly following our clear directives. Once we send our soldiers into war, we have an obligation to them for the suffering they experience on our behalf.

Klay (2018) raises further the leadership question as to whether our military can sustain "a sense of purpose when nobody . . . seems to take the wars we are fighting seriously?" When civilian leadership fails to articulate "a mission . . . worth dying for . . . soldiers may stop caring about the mission altogether" (72). Klay suggests they stop fighting for the ill-defined mission and rather fight more for the safety of one another. "But if you think the mission your country keeps sending you on is pointless or impossible and that you're only deploying to protect your brothers and sisters in arms from danger then it's not the Taliban or al-Queda or ISIS that's trying to kill you, it's America" (73). What role do we each play in this problem?

Klay, as well as others, suggest that soldiers experience both physical danger and moral injury. The moral injury is on a microlevel and macrolevel. On a microlevel, soldiers in combat under intense pressure can make moment-to-moment mistakes. On a macrolevel, our country and military command under pressure can make moral mistakes. All these levels are related.

Our continuing response to 9/11 illustrates these interconnections. On a macrolevel, Congress—with little debate and the urging of President Bush—authorized the military to find and bring to justice the perpetrators of the 9/11 attack. According to Christopher Whipple's recent book, *The Gatekeepers*, there was no cabinet level review of the president's decision to invade Iraq. Osama bin Laden was eventually found and killed, an action morally justified by most Americans. The legislation has largely been used to continue a nearly two-decade war against terrorism around the world. Our troops are now deployed in Iraq, Afghanistan, Syria, Yemen, Libya, Somalia, and Niger to name a few places. Callimachi et al. record that there are about 5,000 to 6,000 soldiers in Africa. In contrast, there are 14,000 in Afghanistan, 25,000 in Korea, 35,000 in Germany, and 40,000 in Japan (9).

In retrospect, the war was declared on the basis of information later proven to be incorrect. This error leads to questions about the ability to trust that government will make correct decisions.

The lack of defined purpose and moral clarity of this continuing mission is underscored by the reaction of congressional leaders to the killings of four Green Berets in Niger in the fall of 2017. Both Senators Schumer and Graham acknowledged ignorance of the presence of so many American troops in Niger. Senator Rand Paul said, as stated in *The New York Times*, "What we have today is basically unlimited war—war anywhere, anytime, anyplace on the globe. I don't think anyone with an ounce of intellectual honesty believes these authorizations allow current wars we fight in seven countries."

On a microlevel, these Green Berets were there to provide training and assistance to Nigerian forces and facilitate intelligence gathering. They were performing the typical tasks assigned to a counterinsurgency team trying to "win the hearts and minds" of indigenous people. In October 2017, they engaged in supporting a combat team attempting to gather individuals and information about who had kidnapped an American aid worker. *The New York Times* reported that such a change in mission would likely have had the approval of a chain of command at various locations. These officers by rank could include a major and lieutenant colonel up to the level of a two star general in Germany at the US Africa Command where special operations are managed. Through a series of weather and logistically related matters and command errors, the combat team abandoned their mission, but the Green Berets, there to advise, persisted. They found themselves in a hazardous environment but expected no enemy contact. They were ambushed shortly thereafter, having spent hours giving out medicine to allegedly sick village children. The helicopters, drones, and jet planes that normally accompany combat troops were allegedly not there for this advisory team. These four Green Berets sent to advise and not primarily to fight were killed in combat, in a morally ambiguous situation. Family members are asking who and what are their sons fighting. (Callimachi et al. 9).

These soldiers did not survive. Had they survived, they might well have experienced trauma from lack of safety. They might also have experienced the moral trauma related to the loss of trust in oneself, in one's judgment, in others, the mission, the military, and in the country as a whole.

CHAPTER TWENTY-EIGHT

# THE EFFECT OF QUALITY LEADERSHIP

Physicians have many qualities. Being a natural leader is not always one of them. My experience with the Army has really opened my eyes on this leadership issue. The past medical leader of our unit was full of great ideas, but he lacked focus, efficiency, and a cooperative spirit, which led to fragmented care and demoralized staff.

When our medical leader "disappeared," the Army bureaucracy moved in and took over. Regulations appeared everywhere. There were sign-in and sign-out sheets, multiple time sheets, protocols, and treatment plans. Once "the new rules" were in place, a high-ranking enlisted man was assigned to be our administrative leader. He was the NCOIC, or the noncommissioned officer, in charge. I remembered NCOICs from my Army experience. They are trained to be leaders, and he was arriving to lead us. I decided to watch, listen, and ask questions.

He was young, almost half the age of our "seasoned" medical staff members. He was upbeat and enthusiastic. We surmised that he knew little about behavioral health and psychiatry. We were correct, but he was willing to learn. He thought physicians were poorly prepared to be leaders in the military, and he did not mind expressing his viewpoint. I admit I was "put off" if not offended by this viewpoint. I asked questions, and he was eager to discuss. I learned that he had grown up in a difficult innercity environment. He knew about surviving in "gangs." Deployment in war was safer than being in his neighborhood. He understood how to get individuals to work together. That got my attention.

I knew that competing with one another to get into medical school, surviving the rigors of a medical curriculum, and working 120 hours a week during residency might foster an illusion in us that we physicians can accomplish whatever we determine to tackle. Certainly it creates a sense of self-determination and autonomy. Being in charge of and responsible for oneself, however, is not the same as being in charge of and responsible for others.

"So, why aren't physicians good leaders in the Army?" I asked.

"It starts with the selection process," the NCOIC said (hereafter referred to as our "leader"). "Being curious about biology, thinking in a very reductionist manner, and memorizing reams of data is not training for leadership. It might get you through medical school." I acknowledged so much studying and clinical training was competitive and implemented within a fairly sheltered lifestyle.

The leader went on to compare the training of soldiers and physician officers. By the time a physician officer in the Army is a field grade officer—major or above—he or she has just completed his residency training. Then they are given the command of a unit. Hence, they rise to a command level with no leadership experience. Comparatively, by the time a regularly commissioned officer becomes a major, he or she has had at least two prior combat command positions and passed several performance reviews. Interesting point! I started to pay more attention.

The leader continued, "The law even fosters poor physician leadership." "What do you mean by that?" I asked. Previously, he had been in charge of a unit in which he was unable to terminate a physician who was performing in an incompetent manner. Physicians whose medical training is paid for by the military owe the military future time in service for their prior training. Congress passed a law saying that physicians who are paying back their time cannot be terminated from their jobs. How did this young leader deal with that problem? He discovered that the physician was writing narcotic prescriptions for prostitutes in exchange for services. He could not legally terminate the physician, but he could report illegal behavior. The incompetent physician was no longer a problem for his unit. Good leaders can work around even congressional obstacles, I learned.

I also learned that this leader was not just expressing his own opinion about physicians being unprepared for effective leadership in the military. It is a viewpoint widely held. An unclassified Officer Leader Development Study, published in 2013, reported that physicians accounted for 21 percent of all Army officers. The report's findings showed that this unintended consequence came from the way physicians were recruited and trained in the military. Physician officers are not, the report stated, "adequately . . . inspired, or motivated upon entry into the Army Profession, . . . or adequately developed as leaders through military education, . . . [as their training is] focused more on managing the business of the healthcare system" than leadership.

"So, what if all physicians are not good leaders?" I asked. Our leader spoke directly to the 2009 Fort Hood shootings by physician Maj. Nidal Hassan. Stating that this was just his opinion, of course, he outlined how the prior medical command did not deal with Hassan's obvious problems in his prior assignment. He made the case for the failure of medical leadership being a factor in the Fort Hood shootings. It made me think of the Hippocratic Oath.

So, has the leadership of our new NCOIC made a difference for our psychiatrists? Unquestionably yes. We are clear about what we are doing, we know how to do it, and we can rely on one another. And soldiers can rely on us. Our NCOIC's leadership has made a difference because of the way he facilitated *how* we do what we *know* how to do.

Our leader was so good that a higher-level command ordered him to go elsewhere for another leadership position. We are technically leaderless, but his lingering effects are such that we are doing rather well without a leader. Isn't that the sign of a good leader? Our enhanced effectiveness is a testimony to him, and even more, a "medical benefit" to soldiers.

## PROFESSIONAL REFLECTIONS

The military teaches effective leadership. The military needs physicians. Physicians are not trained to be leaders. Our NCOIC's leadership made a difference. He facilitated *how* we do as an organization what we *know* how to do individually. As private practitioners, we were effective and efficient individual clinicians. As an organization with a charismatic creative former leader, we had many innovative yet inefficient organizational programs.

Our NCOIC imposed regulations everywhere. He determined that our clinical work was not being properly coded for billing purposes. We all went to coding school, learned how to properly administratively code for clinical work, and our billings soared. He also reduced our work force by 80 percent while maintaining 66 percent of the overall productivity. By streamlining our programs, one fifth of our workforce was performing almost as much clinical work as the prior group with five times as many people. We became so successful that the military investigated us, suspecting that we were "cheating" on our billings. He taught us how to do more with less.

If one needs further evidence that physicians are not necessarily good leaders and should be trained to be so, one can examine the case of Maj. Nidal Hassan. Doctor Hassan was the physician Army officer who fatally shot thirteen people and injured thirty-two others at Fort Hood, Texas, in 2009. The implications of his prior public statements were not fully appreciated by both the FBI and his fellow physician officers.

In a large system, just having good physicians does not necessarily lead to quality medical care. The quality of leadership makes a significant difference in the delivery of the medical care. The 2018 political controversy about leadership of the Veterans Administration speaks to this issue.

CHAPTER TWENTY-NINE

# THE VALUE OF LISTENING

## PERSONAL REFLECTION

**The following essay describes an experience I had after my job of working with soldiers was terminated. The story captures what can be the benefit for soldiers and citizens by getting to know one another.**

**Sam was a depressed cancer survivor with an autistic child. He describes the "gift of working with soldiers" and how the accidental experience put his life in perspective. His time, attention, and fundraising for them, his gifts to them, fostered a renewed perspective on his own future. His efforts were difficult but fruitful.**

I went to the gym to exercise. I jumped on a bike equidistant between Fox and CNN. As I glanced at the televisions, the guy next to me was just getting off a cell phone conversation. "Are you a lawyer?" he said. "I'm having trouble with my lawyer." Sam had forgotten that I was a physician. We speak only occasionally but never fail to say hello. "Oh, yeah, forgot. I get along with all my physicians," he continued.

"My doctor thinks I am depressed and that I am in denial."

"What makes them think that?" I rather automatically responded.

"I had stage IV incurable cancer, had a few months to live, and the radiation closed off one of my coronary arteries," he replied. He had my attention. Knowing I had seen him almost daily for several years, I asked, "How long ago was the cancer?"

"About ten years," he said.

"Sounds like you should be thankful not depressed," I said.

"It changed my life," he exclaimed.

I knew from various anecdotes over the years that Sam was a very tough guy. He grew up on the streets of New York. He was exceptionally good with his hands and was an expert in martial arts. At age five, his father put him on the street corner and challenged anyone to fight him. As an adult civilian, he taught hand-to-hand combat to Navy SEALs and Special Forces. With a little prodding, he admitted that he could "take" most soldiers but by the end he was always exhausted and they were not even sweating. He knew that if you put a gun in a soldier's hands he was a dead man despite his superior hand-to-hand skills.

After high school, Sam worked in the street in "collections." One day, he was collecting money from local businesses and some kids reported a body in a car. Some people thought he was just sleeping there, but when the EMTs arrived he was as stiff as a board. The man was either frozen or in rigor mortis. From across the street, Sam observed the kids throwing bottles and cans at the body. Shocked, he said to himself, "I have to get off the street or within a few years that could be me."

"So, how did the cancer change your life?" I asked.

"I'm Catholic, so I decided to go to see a priest in confession," he said. "I told him I had most of the commandments covered, but I had one fault. Whenever I talked with Christ, I always treated Him as an equal. I am really an arrogant SOB. The priest asked me what have I ever done for one person. I had no answer. That's when I decided to dedicate 20 percent of my time volunteering with soldiers.

"I work with a buddy who started an organization that takes soldiers from Walter Reed to dinner one night a week. We dine with the guys with two and three amputations. I told the soldiers from the beginning that I was a no-sympathy-type guy, and they seem all right with that. I look them in the eye the entire time, but it is really hard to keep your eyes off their prostheses. Finally, I decided to just talk to them about it and it changed everything. I discovered that once they get over the mental problem of having lost a limb or two, they can function just like me. We even play in golf tournaments together."

Sam further explained how he helped found a home-building program for veterans. Their home purchasing program received great publicity, and they now produce one home for a veteran's family every ten days all over the United States. He was surprised at the difficulty of dealing with some spouses. They fuss over the marble countertops in the kitchen. "It's free," he said. But over time, after realizing they are the real caretakers for the rest of a soldier's life, he became more tolerant. Sam also recounted how he grew up with "a little OCD" and worried about his health. Now, he has had cancer and a child with autism. The gift of working with soldiers has put that all in perspective. "I just deal with it, without feeling sorry for myself," he said.

Sam said he worked all right with amputees, but he didn't really understand PTSD and traumatic brain injury. He had childhood friends who had each killed more than two or three people and said it was just their job. They did not seem troubled. But he mused, "I am told war is 90 percent boredom and 10 percent absolute terror and fear." He recounted his time with Tony, who has PTSD. In the middle of the conversation, as he was looking directly into his eyes, Tony just seemed to disappear and be in another place. Sam did not know what to do. Tony spent a couple of months in a mental hospital, but now he is back with the group.

Sam recounted another occasion after Tony had returned from deployment. An accident brought him to a civilian hospital where he was treated. His family received a large hospital bill. Veterans have no civilian health insurance upon returning from deployment. Sam thought it was outrageous and should be the next day's headlines in *The Washington Post*. He said everyone would be equally outraged, but the next day the "news" would be forgotten. He agreed that more civilians need to know about the problems of veterans.

As Sam was walking away, I heard him say, "I used to believe in war. Now, I just don't know."

## CHAPTER THIRTY

# A LONG GOODBYE

Rumored for years, long anticipated, yet sudden in arrival, and sobering when it happened, the US Army announced that our civilian contract to provide medical services to veterans and current servicemen and women would not be renewed. I felt simultaneously angry and liberated. Angry that I had to stop providing a service that had given me so much. Liberated because I knew at some level, I might not have been able stop on my own. In retrospect, these nearly eight years of providing medication and psychotherapy to service members and their families has been an unexpected gift, a capstone to over fifty years in a medical career.

In 2009, I was intrigued by a medical recruiter's phone call offering a position in the Department of Psychiatry at the Walter Reed Army Medical Center. Working as a government-employed psychiatrist offered tantalizing retirement possibilities. Seeing patients in remote locations via closed circuit television, telehealth seemed unusual, but I decided to look further. The application and security clearance process was onerous. Credentialing approval at a dozen Army installations was long and tedious. Training courses and learning to use electronic medical records taxed my brain. But the "trappings" were inspiring.

The Walter Reed campus, the location of the telehealth services, was more than 100 years old. Uniformed men and women are exceedingly polite and gracious. The weekly helicopter landing with evacuees is mesmerizing. Watching the servicemen with multiple amputations negotiate the cafeteria with their wives and children or girlfriends is something every American should see. I have to admit I was smitten.

By providing medical services, we were with the military but not in the military. We provided the service virtually (closed circuit television) to them, but it was a vicarious experience for us. Their altruism is infectious. Paradoxically, the virtual experience allowed us to get closer to the service members. They knew that they and their secrets would not meet us later in the PX or on their base. The physical distance allowed more emotional candor.

By 2010, the telehealth department had fifteen years of experience providing service to locations outside of the United States. Before my arrival, the leader had decided to develop a virtual MTF or military training facility. The service grew from five people to more than seventy with psychiatrists, psychologists, social workers, neurologists, neurosurgeons, nurse practitioners, physician assistants, physical therapists, occupational therapists, and dermatologists with locations across the country. There were many ongoing research projects.

Our telehealth service was growing. But so was Walter Reed, which was in the midst of a transition from its historic location to the new facility combined with the Navy. Unfortunately, our charismatic leader, who allegedly got direct funding from Congress and the "powers that be" at Walter Reed, did not allocate sufficient space for our service in the transition to the new Walter Reed location. They left, and we were left in the old location that was closing.

Finding an electronically secure building approved by the Department of Defense is complicated. Eventually, the logistical problem was resolved by a move to a secure building near the

Pentagon. We moved into a floor that seemed the size of a football field. The space was too big for our current staff but large enough for our anticipated growth.

In finding a place, the logistics were one thing, but finding an administrative home was another. We worked well clinically and administratively within our unit, but we were not administratively connected to the larger military service. We provided clinical service all over the United States. But not fitting into a TOE, someone's Table of Organization and Equipment, and not being "owned" by a higher level military institution may have been our undoing. We were "rogues," but we clinicians were oblivious to the administrative issue.

We survived many problems on our journey. When the government was shut down in October 2013, our service was suspended. Later, a failure to get the civilian contracts in order put us out of work for three to four weeks. One day, to everyone's surprise, our leader was escorted off the premises by armed military guards. It was tense, but we created a space for our own support. Nevertheless, these disturbances led some of the younger professionals to seek more "stable" employment.

New leadership thought we were insufficiently productive. It is called not enough "billable hours." We thought we were working very hard. An investigation revealed that our work was not being properly coded; hence, it looked as if we were not doing enough work. Coding workshops and an onsite coder remedied that problem. Armed with coding expertise, we continued our work. Shortly thereafter, we became, on paper, the most efficient productive unit in military telehealth. "They" thought we were cheating, so another investigation ensued. The conclusion: Proper coding showed that we were in fact doing that much work.

Leadership changed again, and an effort to close our unit ensued. It became politically impossible because our service was deemed so essential to the various sites around the country. This type of stress yields attrition. Gradually, providers sought other jobs. Our provider numbers declined. Finally, the sudden, really unexpected, announcement arrived. The civilian contract would not be renewed. A telehealth service, firmly administratively ensconced at another military post, would replace us. The date was set. More providers left.

Now, near the end, there are three psychiatrists remaining. We have over 1,000 patients among us. We are saying "goodbye" to each and everyone one of them. How does one explain the above story? Yet, every one of these service members "gets it." They know how a large bureaucracy works. They know these decisions are often made by individuals who never see "patients."

We three psychiatrists have more than 150 years of clinical experience and over twenty-five years of experience in telehealth. None of that makes the goodbyes any easier. These eight years have been a gift.

# PART VIII

# AFTERWORD

CHAPTER THIRTY-ONE

# STORIES FROM OUTSIDE OUR MORAL UNIVERSE

## PERSONAL REFLECTION

This essay presents a view of war and its physical and moral trauma.

***"Never think that war no matter how necessary nor how justified is not a crime. Ask the infantry and ask the dead. No weapon has ever settled a moral problem. It can impose a solution but it cannot guarantee it to be a just one. You can wipe out your opponents. But if you do it unjustly you become eligible for being wiped out yourself."***

**—(Hemingway, Introduction to *Treasury for the Free World,* 1946)**

Civilians live in a conventional moral universe with rules of behavior dictated—among other things—by the Bible, the Koran, the Declaration of Independence, and the United States Constitution.

They learn the golden rule of doing "unto others what you want done unto yourself." They know the prohibition against killing, learn about the common good, and proclaim a country united by a common creed.

Soldiers do not operate within this universe. Soldiers exist in a combat space, a universe that disregards our conventional moral one. They learn of "just wars" that set out rules of engagement—the end game is to kill the enemy. These rules are highly technical and instructive and, as such, give legitimacy to this space. They include proportionality in how to fight, how long to fight, and with whom to fight and kill. This universe brings with it a morality profoundly at odds with our conventional one.

The soldier's bible is the "Infantry Rifle Platoon and Squad" field manual, 340 pages long. It sets aside conventional morality by graphically describing the primary role of a soldier. Infantry war "is close combat . . . characterized by extreme violence and physiological shock," which "is callous and unforgiving." This universe is measured in minutes and meters, and its consequences are final. The field manual describes "every aspect of the physical, mental and spiritual standards that count most in battle. Recruits are carefully selected, trained and deployed to meet or exceed these dimensions" (3-21.8). In this way, war turns conventional morality upside down by asking soldiers to deny life, liberty, and property to others. Actions considered clearly criminal in the civilian moral universe are condoned in the moral universe of combat.

With this new moral compass, soldiers grapple with questions of life, death, and responsibility in this combat space. Although the rules of engagement are thorough and detailed, the application of these guidelines is complicated and fraught with error. In the fog of war, ambiguous circumstances arise, increasing the possibility of making mistakes. Incorrect decisions are made. The wrong people are killed. Women and children and noncombatants are maimed or murdered. Circumstances of battle sometimes make it impossible to help them. They cannot always protect a buddy from the same fate. Witnessing intense suffering combined with the fatigue of battle can lead to anger, guilt, and revengeful acts. Lacking time to grieve, soldiers say "don't get sad, get even."

Soldiers become aware that in the heat of battle they can engage in behavior that is "evil" by any standard. Needless killing of an enemy can perversely make up for the loss of a buddy. Sometimes, behaviors violate not only the civilian moral codes but the combat moral codes. They can enter into spaces not previously imagined.

Humanity has learned that the exploration of new spaces results in new viewpoints. Columbus explored geographic space, and Magellan circumnavigated the world, and humanity learned that the earth was no longer flat but spherical. Astronauts explored physical space, looking back at earth from outerspace, which permitted a new view of the world within the universe. These journeys have been difficult but generally positive. Soldiers move from one moral universe to another in which the rules of behavior have been turned upside down. They also return from this unimagined moral universe with a different mindset and not always a positive one.

While engaging in what was previously morally repugnant behavior, their lives, personal networks, and moral self-images are changed. They arrive back home scarred and self-questioning. In addition to repairing their physical and psychological wounds, there must be an internal reckoning of their moral trauma. The adjustment is profound and difficult.

While citizens are not directly responsible for the soldiers' combat experiences, citizens do have a responsibility to help with the suffering experienced by these men and women who served in our place. Citizens have the responsibility to help remediate the physical, psychological, and moral suffering experienced by these, our proxies.

Citizen responsibilities are both institutional and personal. The Veterans Administration network of hospitals and outpatient medical centers provides an institutional response. Despite obvious difficulties of a large bureaucracy, the VA works comprehensively and creatively. Physical trauma repair and rehabilitation by the VA and the Army are remarkable and instructive. Their prototypes readily and successfully benefit civilian trauma programs. Civilian trauma directly benefits from the lessons learned in treating warrior trauma.

The personal citizen responsibility to returning warriors has been recognized for centuries. Ancient Greeks publicly performed tragic plays to dramatize the moral traumas experienced in the Trojan War. The Greeks understood that some moral trauma was too severe to be processed individually but needed to be part of a community experience. This shared civilian and warrior experience led to a collective processing of the grief associated with war.

How can we personally assist our veterans? The answer rests in our awareness and resulting action. The military has identified two routes to moral repair—one involving emotions and one involving acceptance. The emotional route involves telling one's story, one's experience in war. This route requires the speaker to self-regulate in accordance with the situation and the listener to be able to hear what seems "unhearable." Skilled mental health professionals working with soldiers have developed psychotherapy techniques to facilitate this process. Additional research suggests that, subsequently, citizens who are able "to listen" can also help. There are multiple opportunities in book clubs, libraries, schoolrooms, town meetings, churches, synagogues, and YMCAs for citizens to listen.

The second route involves the moral repair of being accepted back into the civilian moral universe. Having engaged in "necessary criminal behavior," a soldier must make peace with himself back home while finding acceptance among us. These individuals who have witnessed or performed mortal atrocities must be able to find redemption within themselves and in our midst. Within our moral universe they must find and experience a sense of goodness. Good people sometimes do awful things and must find a way to live with it and beyond it. Veterans who cannot find their way commit suicide every day at an alarming rate. We owe them the opportunity to share in their moral grief. Frequent acts of kindness are effective.

Sharing in the soldier's moral grief is not just a national duty; rather, it is a moral obligation that citizens owe to soldiers who fought in their place. There are benefits. Knowing soldiers and their experiences is an extraordinary opportunity. It seems counterintuitive to confront trauma and find peace, to see death and find life, to experience paralysis and find choice, or to experience loss and find connection. Knowing a soldier personally is perhaps the most powerful intervention of all. It goes beyond treating him or her as a hero by thanking him for his service or saluting him at a baseball game. It involves an ongoing connection with that soldier, his family, or his orphan and to hear and witness to how he or she pieces a life back together again. That soldier's struggle will enlighten your struggle and your journey. It is a reciprocal relationship. We owe it to one another. They went to war in our place and now we must welcome them back to our home. It is important to the future of our society—for all that divides us—that we collectively witness their narrative.

If you have any doubt about the transformative effect of listening to soldiers, turn to the life and poetry of Walt Whitman, arguably America's greatest poet. Visiting and listening to thousands of soldiers during the America Civil War, he "saved himself" by describing the experience as "the greatest privilege and satisfaction of (my) life." By listening to their stories, there is no guarantee you will become a poet, but you will become a more mature and informed adult. America needs you.

# CITATIONS

"The American Veterans' and Service Members' Survival Guide." http://www.nvisp.org/images/Survival%20Guide-102309.pdf. Accessed 20 June 2018.

Amidon, Amy. "Healing a Wounded Sense of Morality." *The Atlantic.* 3 July 2015. www.theatlantic.com. Accessed 20 June 2018.

Armstrong, Keith, Suzanne Best, and Paula Domenici. "Tips for Getting Better Sleep." *Courage After Fire: Coping Strategies for Troops Returning from Iraq and Afghanistan and Their Families.* 2006

Ballenger-Browning K.K., K.J. Schmitz, J.A. Rothacker, et al. "Predictors of Burnout Among Military Mental Health Providers." *Military Medicine.* 176:253–260, 2011. Web. Accessed 20 June 2018.

Beah, Ishmael. *A Long Way Gone: Memoirs of a Boy Soldier*. Sarah Crichton Books, 2008.

Berkson, Mark, PhD. "Denial of Death, Dying and the Afterlife." *The Great Courses.* Department of Religion Hamline University Lecture. www.thegreatcourses.com/ Accessed 20 June 2018.

Bolger, Dan. *Why We Lost: A General's Inside Account of the Iraq and Afghanistan Wars*. Houghton Mifflin Harcourt, 2014.

Brennan, Thomas J. USMC (Ret) and Finbarr O'Reilly. *Shooting Ghosts A U.S. Marine, A Combat Photographer, and Their Journey Back from War*. Viking Press, 2017.

Brooks, David. "The Moral Injury." *New York Times.* 17 February 2015. www.nytimes.com/2015/02/17/opinion/david-brooks-the-moral-injury.html. Accessed 20 June 2018.

Bush, George W. "Military Service Initiative, Veteran Transition." George W. Bush Institute. www.bushcenter.org.

Bush, George W. *Portraits of Courage: A Commander in Chief's Tribute to America's Warriors.* Crown Publisher/Random House, 2017.

Callimachi, Rukmini, Helene Cooper, Eric Schmitt, Alan Blinder, and Thomas Gibbons-Neff. "A Risky Patrol, A Desert Ambush and New Anguish Over 'An Endless War.' " *New York Times*. Sunday 18 February 2018, p.1.

Candler, Pete. "I Wish I Had the Courage to Ask My Dad about His Service in Vietnam." *The Washington Post.* 10 November 2017. www.washingtonpost.com/outlook/i-wish-i-had-the-courage-to-ask-my-dad-about-his-service-in-vietnam/2017/11/09/a2af3090-c4a8-11e7-afe9-4f60b5a6c4a0_story.html?utm_term=.71217d4b1807. Accessed 20 June 2018.

Danzig, Richard and Peter Szanton. *National Service: What Would It Mean?* Lexington Books, 1986.

Doerries, Bryan. *Theater of War: What Ancient Tragedies Can Teach Us Today.* Vintage, 2016.

"Escaping the Grip of PTSD." *Dartmouth Medicine.* Fall 2013, pp. 38-43. http://dartmed.dartmouth.edu/fall13/html/ptsd/. Accessed 20 June 2018.

"The Face of Battle, Americans at War, 9/11 to Now." *National Portrait Gallery.* 7 April 2017-28 January 2018. http://npg.si.edu/exhibition/face-battle-americans-war-911-now. Accessed 20 June 2018.

Eltagouri, Marwa. "This Fighter Pilot Flew the Last Mission over Japan in WWII. Then He Learned to Love His Enemy." *The Washington Post.* 7 December 2017. www.washingtonpost.com/news/retropolis/wp/2017/12/07/jerry-yellin-flew-the-last-mission-over-japan-in-wwii-then-he-learned-to-love-his-enemy/?utm_term=.df569337faf9. Accessed 20 June 2018.

Fallows, James. "The Draft: Why the Country Needs It." *The Atlantic.* April 1980. www.theatlantic.com/magazine/archive/2015/01/the-tragedy-of-the-american-military/383516/. Accessed 20 June 2018.

Fallows, James. "The Tragedy of the American Military." *The Atlantic.* January/February 2015. www.theatlantic.com/magazine/archive/2015/01/the-tragedy-of-the-american-military/383516/. Accessed 20 June 2018.

Field, Kimberly C. "Veterans, Be Thankful for Your Service." *The Washington Post.* 24 November 2017. www.highbeam.com/publications/the-washington-post-p5554/nov-24-2017. Accessed 20 June 2018.

Goodman, H.A. "6,845 Americans Died and 900,000 Were Injured in Iraq and Afghanistan. Say 'No' to Obama's War." *Huffington Post.* 14 April 2015. www.huffingtonpost.com/h-a-goodman/6845-americans-died-and-9_b_6667830.html. Accessed 20 June 2018.

Goodman, H.A. "4,486 American Soldiers Have Died in Iraq. President Obama Is Continuing a Pointless and Deadly Quagmire." *Huffington Post.* 6 December 2017. www.huffingtonpost.com/h-a-goodman/4486-american-soldiers-ha_b_5834592.html. Accessed 20 June 2018.

Hoge, C.W., C.G. Ivany, and A. B. Adler. "Suicidal Behaviors Within Army Units: Contagion and Implications for Public Health Interventions." *JAMA Psychiatry.* 2017-74(9):871-872. https://www.ncbi.nlm.nih.gov/pubmed/28746711. Accessed 20 June 2018.

Ignatius, David. "At Last, Afghans on the Front Lines." *The Washington Post.* 9, January 2018.

"The Infantry Rifle Platoon and Squad," Field Manual FM 3-21.8 (FM7-8). Headquarters No. 3-21.8 Department of the Army Washington, DC, 28 March 2007. Commandant, USAIS, ATTN: ATSH-ATD, 675.1 www.utm.edu/departments/milsci/_pdfs/FM%203-21.8_Infantry%20Rifle%20Platoon%20and%20Squad.pdf. Accessed 20 June 2018.

Jackson J. Mark. "Another Perspective: A Veteran's Dark Lifetime Gift." *The Washington Post* 17 November 2018. http://www.newschief.com/opinion/20171117/another-perspective-veterans-dark-lifetime-gift. Accessed 20 June 2018.

Junger, Sebastian. *Tribe: On Homecoming and Belonging.* Twelve, Hachette Book Group, 2016.

Junger, Sebastian. *War.* Twelve, Hachette Book Group, 2010.

Khan, Amat and Anand Gopal. "The Uncounted." *The New York Times Magazine.* 16 November 2017. www.nytimes.com/interactive/2017/11/16/magazine/uncounted-civilian-casualties-iraq-airstrikes.html. Accessed 20 June 2017.

Killebrew, R. "What Others Are Saying." *Chicago Tribune.* 13 November 2017.

Klay, Phil. "The Warrior at the Mall." *Sunday Review, New York Times.* 15 April 2018.

Klay, Phil. *Redeployment.* Penguin Group, 2014.

Klein, Joe. *Charlie Mike: A True Story of Heroes Who Brought Their Mission Home.* Simon & Schuster, 2015.

Lamothe, Dan. "Brothers in Arms." *The Washington Post Letters from War.* 6 December 2017. https://www.washingtonpost.com/graphics/2017/national/world-war-two-letters/?utm_term=.f895e2925fd7. Accessed 20 June 2018.

Levin, Aaron. "STARRS Findings Shed More Light on Army Suicides." *Psychiatric News.* Published Online:14 May 2018. https://doi.org/10.1176/appi.pn.2018.5b19. Accessed 20 June 2018.

MacLeish, Archibald. "The Young Dead Soldiers Do Not Speak."

Mason, Wyatt. "Homer's Daughter." *The New York Times Magazine.* 2 November 2017. www.nytimes.com/2017/11/02/magazine/the-first-woman-to-translate-the-odyssey-into-english.html. Accessed 20 June 2018.

MacGregor, Jeff. "The Healing Power of Greek Tragedy." *Smithsonian.com.* November 2017, pp. 75-98. https://www.smithsonianmag.com/arts-culture/healing-power-greek-tragedy-180965220/. Accessed 20 June 2018.

McPherson, James M. *Abraham Lincoln and the Second American Revolution.* Oxford University Press, 1992.

Meacham, John. "A Year that Made the Present Seem Tranquil." *Time.* 29 January 2018, p.19. www.magzter.com. Accessed 20 June 2018.

Mendelsohn, Daniel. *An Odyssey: A Father, A Son and an Epic.* Alfred A. Knopf, 2017.

Moran, Mark. "Military Has Lessons to Share with Medicine." *Psychiatric News.* 17 November 2017, p.1. psychnews.psychiatryonline.org. Accessed 20 June 2018.

"More about the Brain." Appendix C: *Resilience 101: Understanding and Optimizing Your Stress System.* Pamela Woll, MA CADP. www.scribd.com/document/37399860/Resilience-101-Workbook. Accessed 20 June 2018.

Nagel, Thomas (1979). "Moral Luck" (PDF). *Mortal Questions.* Cambridge: Cambridge University Press, 2012. pp. 24–38. OCLC 4135927. www.cambridge.org. Accessed 20 June 2018.

Nasr, Suhayl. "No Laughing Matter; Laughter Is Good Psychiatric Medicine." *Current Psychiatry.* 2013 August. 12(8):20-25. /www.mdedge.com/psychiatry/article/76797/bipolar-disorder/no-laughing-matter-laughter-good-psychiatric-medicine. Accessed 20 June 2018.

"Performance in Practice: Clinical Tools to Improve the Care of Patients with Posttraumatic Stress disorder." *FOCUS: The Journal of Lifelong Learning in Psychiatry.* Spring 2009 Vol. VII no. 2 p 186-203. focus.psychiatryonline.org/doi/10.1176/foc.7.2.foc186. Accessed 20 June 2018.

"Preventing Vicarious Trauma: What Counselors Should Know When Working with Trauma Survivors." Trippany, R.L. *Journal of Counseling & Development.* Winter 2004. Vol 82:31.

"Prevention of Posttraumatic Stress Disorder by Early Treatment: Results from the Jerusalem Trauma Outreach and Prevention Study." *Arch Gen Psychiatry.* Wol69 (no.2). Feb. 2012. www.ncbi.nlm.nih.gov. Accessed 20 June 2018.

Raddatz, Martha. *The Long Road Home: A Story of War and Family.* Berkley Trade, 2008.

Reich, Robert B. *The Common Good.* New York: Alfred A. Knopf, 2018.

"Repeat Brain Injury Raises Soldiers' Suicide Risk." *Science Daily.* http://www.sciencedaily.com/releases/2013/05/130515163924.htm. Accessed 20 June 2018.

Ricks, Thomas E. "Death Trap: Why So Many Veterans Kill Themselves?" *Chicago Tribune.* 6 April 2018. https://www.sltrib.com/opinion/commentary/2018/04/

Scurfield, Ray DSW. "War Trauma Resources." http://www.usm.edu/socialwork/scurfield/Index.php. Accessed 20 June 2018.

Shay, Jonathan. *Achilles in Vietnam: Combat Trauma and the Undoing of Character.* Scribner, 1994.

Shay, Jonathan. *Odysseus in America: Combat Trauma and the Trials of Homecoming.* Scribner, 2002.

Sherman, Nancy. "Hidden Wounds." *Psychology Today.* 29 May 2012. www.psychologytoday.com. Accessed 20 June 2018.

Sherman, Nancy. *Afterwar: Healing the Moral Wounds of Our Soldiers.* New York: Oxford University Press, 2015.

Sherman, Nancy. *The Untold War: Inside the Hearts, Minds and Souls of Our Soldiers.* W.W. Norton, 2011.

Sloan, Denise M, Brian P. Marx, Daniel J. Lee, et al. "A Brief Exposure-Based Treatment vs Cognitive Processing Therapy for Posttraumatic Stress Disorder: A Randomized Noninferiority Clinical Trial." *JAMA Psychiatry.* 2018:75(3):233-239. Accessed 20 June 2018.

Smith, Harrison. "British Surgeon Who Treated Both Sides in the Falklands War." *The Washington Post.* 17 January 2018. www.washingtonpost.com/local/obituaries/rick-jolly-british-navy-surgeon-who-treated-both-sides-in-falklands-war-dies-at-71/2018/01/16/f826d4d8-facc-11e7-a46b-a3614530bd87_story.html?utm_term=.1d63517021d5. Accessed 20 June 2018.

Steinhorn, Leonard. *The Greater Generation: In Defense of The Baby Boomer Legacy.* Thomas Dunne Books, St. Martin's Press, 2006.

Tennyson, Alfred L. "The Charge of the Light Brigade." *The Examiner.* 9 December 1854. popularvictorianpoetry.wordpress.com. Accessed 20 June 2018.

Ursano, Robert. J. MD., Ronald C. Kessler, PhD., James A. Naifeh, PhD., et al. "Associations of Time-related Deployment Variables with Risk of Suicide Attempt Among Soldiers." Results from the Army Study to Assess Risk and Resilience in Service Members (Army STARRS). *JAMA Psychi*atry. 2018:75(6):596-604. Accessed 20 June 2018.

Ursano, Robert J. MD., Ronald C. Kessler, PhD., and James P. Naifeh, PhD. "Risk of Suicide Attempt Among Soldiers in Army Units With a History of Suicide Attempts." *JAMA Psychiatry.* 2017-74(9):924-931doi:10.1001/jamapsychiatry.2017.1925.

"Veterans Statistics: PTSD, Depression, TBI, Suicide." Veterans and PTSD. 20 September 2015. http://www.veteransandptsd.com/PTSD-statistics.html. Accessed 20 June 2018.

Webb, James. "The Draft: Why the Army Needs It." *The Atlantic Ideas Tour.* April 1980. www.theatlantic.com. Accessed 20 June 2018.

Whipple, Christopher. *Gatekeepers: How the White House Chiefs of Staff Define Every Presidency.* Crown Publishing, 2017.

Will, George. "The Second-most Dangerous American." *The Washington Post.* 23 March 2018. www.washingtonpost.com/opinions/the-second-most-dangerous-american/2018/03/23/90751d80-2ec6-11e8-8688-e053ba58f1e4_story.html?utm_term=.8e3f0765a225. Accessed 20 June 2018.

Williams, Bernard. (1981). "Moral Luck." Moral Luck: Philosophical Papers 1973-1980. Cambridge: Cambridge University Press. pp. 20–39. OCLC 7597880. www.cambridge.org. Accessed 20 June 2018.

Wright, James. *Enduring Vietnam: An American Generation and Its War,* Thomas Dunne Books/St. Martin's Press, April 2017

Zarembo, Alan, David Zucchino, and Molly Hennessy-Fiske. "Fort Hood Shooting Underscores Army's Mental Health Crisis." 4 April 2014. *Los Angeles Times.* http://articles.latimes.com/2014/apr/04/nation/la-na-nn-ft-hood-ptsd-20140404 . Accessed 20 June 2018.

# ACKNOWLEDGMENTS

These essays were written because courageous soldiers stepped forward to seek treatment for their personal response to their war experiences. Without their courage these experiences would never have seen the light of day. Their sacrifice is a gift I will forever cherish.

My wife, Kathleen, encouraged me to write about my encounters with them as a way to gain some perspective on what I was hearing. She read and made insightful and encouraging comments on everything I wrote.

The more I tried to write about what I was hearing, the better I learned to listen. Joe and Mary Ellen Bradley, coeditors and publishers of the *Catholic Peace Fellowship Newsletter*, encouraged me to submit the essays for their publication. Ann Redpath, my ever-faithful editor, tirelessly edited and encouraged the project. Phyllis Theroux, friend and author, encouraged my journal writing and by extension these essays. Her husband, Ragan Phillips, a Naval Academy graduate, read many of the essays and offered constructive suggestions.

As the essays grew in number, they all suggested a book. Ann Redpath continued to edit the essays and offer suggestions such as the introduction, point of view, and the personal reflections. Kathy

Megyeri was an early, frequent, and enthusiastic proponent of the book project, with suggestions from start to finish. "Friends from Chautauqua" Margaret and Michael Kirby, Mary and Tim Gorman, Ginny Daily, and Larry and Janice Pifer were all supportive and encouraging. Larry read the entire book at its inception and was most supportive and encouraging. Allie and Bob Mulvihill were encouraging and helpful in many ways. My wife's book club members were excellent literary critics, especially Jane Lieberthal, who read the entire book and offered her expertise. Scotty Hargrove and Barbara and Paul Wilson were readers of early drafts.

Dartmouth College classmates offered time and constructive criticism. Richard Hannah and John Clarke were especially encouraging. Frank and Dorothy Kehl were early readers and commenters. Frank helped design a public relations campaign, and he and Dorothy attended presentations and offered critiques. David deWilde had insightful comments. Both Craig Dorman and Bill Carpenter read the book and offered comments. David Feingold and Rich Barber added publicity suggestions. James Wright, President Emeritus and Eleazar Wheelock Professor of History Emeritus, at Dartmouth agreed to review the manuscript and comment.

Mark Shields' frequent comments on PBS about the forgotten 1 percent (service members and their families) were always a source of inspiration. John Engels has been an enthusiastic supporter of my work and offered a broad perspective on the importance of the service members' message. Pat Meyer, who has sent her son to war several times, was always faithful to the effort. Susan Luff offered me many opportunities to speak to others about the work. The faculty from The Bowen Center for the Study of the Family/Georgetown Family Center and the faculty from The Center for Family Process have provided many opportunities to speak about the work and receive helpful feedback.

Elaine Rendler, editor of *Today's Liturgy*, was particularly helpful in developing ideas about forgiveness and publishing one of the essays in her magazine. Artist Birdie McElroy was very helpful regarding cover design. Mary Grace Rook, whose son is now deployed in Afghanistan, was an early reader and supporter.

There were many others who helped with ideas about distribution and publicity. Kent Hutchinson and Jim Weiskopf were enormously helpful. Tim Gorman, Heather and Peter Cooke, and Kevin and Angel Magnum and Robert Koffman all agreed to assist with publicity. Miles Irving, Steve Epstein, Don Mellman, Bob Patrick, Richard Hunt, Liza Gold, Alex Rodriguez, Gregory Maggs, Jay Shore, Robert Gallucci, J. R. Quirk, Dennis Laich, Lawrence Wilkerson, Rick Barton, Elspeth Cameron Ritchie, and Henry Sondheimer agreed to offer comments. Lee Cole-Chu was extraordinarily resourceful and helpful in this project. Mary Beth Beal had excellent suggestions. Ann and Kent Cooper were helpful with editing and publicity. Kate Redpath designed a website, and she and Maryalice Beal were very helpful with social media. A special thank you to Bob Dole.

# REFERENCES

Understanding wars required significant reading and research. Below are some of the books I consulted.

*Love My Rifle More Than You* by Kayla Williams and M. Staub; *Band Of Sisters: American Women at War* by Kirsten Holmstedt; *Undaunted: The Real Story of American Service Women* by Tanya Biank and Mark Thompson; *Redeployment* by Phil Klay; *It's My Country Too: Women's Military Stories from the American Revolution to Afghanistan* by Tracy Crown and Jerri Bell; *Shooting Ghosts* by Tom Brennan and Finbarr O'Reilly; *Why We Lost: Generals Insider Account* by Dan Bolger; *Short Like a Girl:One Woman's Dramatic Fight in Afghanistan and the Home Front* by Mary J. Hegar; *The Invisible Front: Love and Loss in an Era of Endless War* by Yochi Dreazen; *Knife Fights: A Memoir of Modern War* by John Nagi.

*Searching for Stars on an Island in Maine* by Alan Lightman; *Run, Don't Walk: The Curious and Courageous Life Inside Walter Reed Army Medical Center* by A. Levine; *Matterhorn* by Karl Marlantes; *Odysseus in*

*America* and *Achilles in Vietnam* by Jonathan Shay; *The Things They Carried* by Tim O'Brien.

*The Long Road Home* by Martha Raddatz; *After Combat: True War Stories from Iraq and Afghanistan* by Marian Eide & Michael Gibler; E*nduring Vietnam: An American Generation and Its War* by James Wright; *365 Days* by Ronald J. Glasser

# WALTER REED ARMY MEDICAL CENTER TELEHEATH ROSTER

Our telehealth service was physically stationed in Washington, DC, at the Walter Reed Army Medical Center in the Department of Psychiatry. It served as a separate virtual outpatient clinic. The section provided a full range of psychiatric services from Walter Reed via secure closed circuit television to the following locations: Aberdeen Proving Ground, Maryland; Fort Belvoir, Virginia; Fort Bragg, North Carolina; Carlisle Barracks, Pennsylvania; Fort Detrick, Maryland; Fort Drum, New York; Fort Hood, Texas; Fort Knox, Tennessee; Fort Lee, Virginia; Fort Meade, Maryland; Pax River Naval Air Station, Maryland; Fort Riley, Kansas; and West Point, New York. Our providers were credentialed at all these locations.

The chairman of the Department of Psychiatry was John C. Bradley, COL MIL USA MEDCOM WRAMC. The head of telepsychiatry was Michael D. Lynch, PhD, ABPP. Initially, Wendy Baynard was our project manager, Adrian King the IT specialist, Deborah Knowles, our nurse case manager, Linda McKnight, Linda Youngblood Sales, and Chery Youngblood Sales, our health system specialists.

Telehealth services and staff expanded rapidly. Our adult psychiatrists included Andrea Adiaconitei, MD; Navneet Atwal,

MD; Edward Beal, MD; Ann C Birk, MD; Christine Daily, MD; Azra Farooqui, MD; Jennifer Park, MD; William Polk, MD; Dianne Reynolds, MD; Paul van Ravenswaay, MD; Lisa Sloat, MD; and Robin Toler, MD. Our child psychiatry staff included Raymond Emanuel, MD, Janice Hutchinson, MD, and Iman Hypolite, MD.

The psychologists included Adam Epstein, PhD; Michael Lynch, PhD; Jauffmick Michel, PsyD; Laura Moulton, PsyD; Jillian Schneider, DVBIC; and Giovanni Scott, PsyD. Our social workers were Ethel Hawkins, LICSW, and Victoria Leonard LCSW. Ann Koons, NP, was our nurse practitioner. Kathleen Ambrose was our TBI program manager. Sharmila Chari, PhD, was our research psychologist. Chistina Yuricevic was our LPN clinical coordinator.

Our service employed personnel at all our remote locations. The author is unable to research the names of all those helpful people but does want to mention Birgit McGill and April Cotter at Aberdeen Proving Ground, Darlene Shughart and Marlene Marsicano at Carlisle Army Barracks, Janice Brown and Annie Kelley at Fort Drum, and Patricia Ranch at Fort Hood.

We experienced transitions in our physical location and in our leadership and administration. When the Walter Reed Army Medical Center moved to Bethesda Naval Medical Center, our group discovered there was not enough physical space for us in Bethesda. We had grown substantially without much notice. When we tried to move thirty-five people to offices for the scheduled four people, we had to find other space. In late 2011, our virtual unit physically moved from Walter Reed Army Medical Center to a secure location near the Pentagon after which Fort Meade and the Department of the Army assumed administrative leadership.

Over the next several years, we moved more than once and added staff and administration. The new administrative members included Angela S. Icaza, LTC; John Sentell, MD; MSG Jason Alexander; Matthew Wills, CPT; Efther Samuel; Simeca Whitener; Janice Cvrk; William Carter; Kenyotta Griffin; Matthew Shogren; and Deanna

Klingensmith. We added further medical staff including Ryan Gorman, NP; Barbara Mazer, PhD; Amanda Trent, PsyD; Shlonda Reed, LPN; Aida Johnson, NP; Evelyn Warner, CAN; Kathryn Wong, speech pathologist; Hanna Sonkey, LPN; La Tonya Gray, RN; Laura Marquart, MD; Dana Lipsky, PsyD; Deanna Little, PsyD, as well as additional administrative staff including Kimberly Johnson, Folashele Olabisi, Kanesha Taylor, Ernest Miller, and Mary Horne.

In August 2017, the telehealth services were administratively transferred to Fort Gordon, Georgia. The circumstances of the transfer are addressed in essay number thirty, "A Long Goodbye."

CPSIA information can be obtained
at www.ICGtesting.com
Printed in the USA
JSHW010707071119
2243JS00001B/1

9 781633 939479